Testimonals

A "LETTER TO MY MOM"

Lisa Hirsch writes with her heart fully open. Her vulnerability and loving approach helps settle rattled souls struggling to find peace with dementia. She engages her readers by exposing her authentic self as she shares her journey with her mother. Lisa teaches people new ways to reframe old thought patterns, helps them find joy and most importantly lets them know they are not alone. I encourage all to read "**LETTER TO MY MOM**."

Lori La Bey
Founder of Alzheimer's Speaks
www.AlzheimersSpeaks.com

If you're looking for a book to take you on the roller coaster ride of caring for a parent with Alzheimer's from a distance, you've found it. I regard Lisa as an expert caregiver in this area and her diary presents the slow progression of this dreaded disease and how she's dealt with it. She reveals her personal insights, fears, sorrows and incredible joys with searing honesty. This new book is telling, heartfelt and heartbreaking—but also intensely life affirming. This is definitely a book that everyone should want to read.
Adrienne Gruberg
Founder and President, The Caregiver Space

Letter To My Mom

Letter To My Mom

My Hero

Alzheimer's -A Daughter's Diary

LISA R. HIRSCH
Book - My Mom My Hero; Alzheimer's
Available from Amazon.com and other retailers

ISBN-13: 9781982071141
ISBN-10: 1982071141
Library of Congress Control Number: 2018900955
CreateSpace Independent Publishing Platform
North Charleston, South Carolina

I Dedicate this Book to my Mother, Ruth Elian, for always loving me and being there for me whether I knew it or not.

As Mother Teresa said,
"We shall never know all the good that a simple smile can do".

Table of Contents

LETTER TO MY MOM
MY HERO
Alzheimer's -A Daughter's Diary

November 2017

It's been over fourteen years that I have been watching my mother's decline from this terrifying disease called Alzheimer's. Mom's younger brother suffered for a few years from this disease before passing away eleven years ago. My grandfather lived to the ripe age of eighty-two and my grandmother died of colon cancer at the age of fifty-six.

Maybe if my grandparents lived longer, especially my grandmother, then they too would have shown signs of dementia. My brother and I wonder what caused this to plague our immediate family. Were there other ancestors who had Alzheimer's?

We have no answer, yet pray that it skips our generation, and those of our children. By then hopefully there will be a cure or at least some prevention.

As I begin sharing my diary with you in this book I would like to give you some history about my mom's life and our mother /daughter relationship.

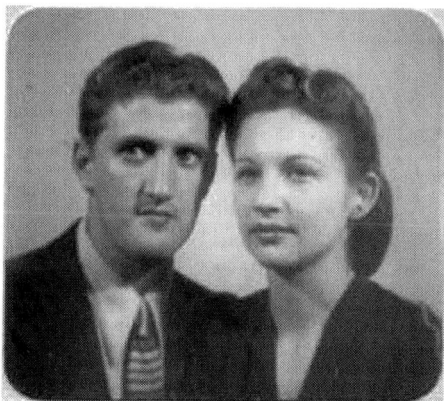

Loving The Mother I Never Knew April, 2011

My mother, Ruth Esther Schnitzer, grew up in Brooklyn and married my father in 1942, when she was just 18 years old. She was blonde, pretty and petite – just under five feet tall – and wore her hair in a pixie cut that suited her feisty personality.

Ruth's father escaped Russia by boat to avoid the persecution of Jews in Europe. He went to work in a sweat shop in New York's garment district, striving to give his children better opportunities than he had. With his encouragement, Ruth loved to read and learn. She continued taking college classes most of her adult life.

My mom gave birth to my brother Gil during World War II when she was 19 years old, and moved in with her parents when my father shipped out with the Navy shortly after that. Mom worked at the military base while my grandmother cared for my brother. When my dad got out of the service, Gil was two years old, and my grandmother and mom were so protective that Dad could hardly have a relationship with him.

Naturally, when I was born five years later, Dad showered me with affection. I adored him as much as he adored me. He was carefree and upbeat, always telling jokes or singing show tunes. He spoiled me, and sometimes I wonder if that's why Mom was so hard on me: maybe she resented me in some way and felt jealous.

In any case, if she'd been one of today's mothers, Ruth would have fallen into the "tough love camp." If I spilled my milk, a quick slap was sure to follow. She was always nervous and ready with a harsh word if you displeased her. Once, for instance, Gil and I gave our parents an electric blanket for an anniversary present, and she immediately said that she didn't like it and was going to return it.

Mom was adamant that I should make the most of myself. She ordered summer reading materials and wouldn't let me out to play until I mastered one lesson every day. I fought those lessons, especially the summer that she handed me particularly difficult assignments that turned out to be for children a grade ahead of me. Mom later bragged about how she made me a better reader by making me study. I felt like I was being tortured and disliked reading for years.

When I was in junior high, we moved to Great Neck, Long Island, an affluent New York suburb. "We want you to better yourself," Mom explained when I cried about leaving our apartment in Queens.

This move was my father's idea, too, of course. He grew up in Manhattan, on the lower East Side, where his father had a pushcart selling vegetables. Dad earned a college degree in accounting and always thought he'd be rich someday. We were never wealthy, but he owned a gas station, a variety store and a tiny factory that made household items sewn by people with disabilities.

Living in this "better" neighborhood made me feel more insecure. I longed for the shoes other girls had – especially the Papagallo shoes in every color – cosmetic surgery to fix my nose, and a grand piano. My mother's favorite word seemed to be "no."

I finally did talk her into getting a dog. Mom brought me to an animal shelter, where we adopted an adorable shaggy, beige-colored dog. I practically ran home every day after school to walk him, I was so thrilled.

And then, one day, the dog wasn't there. Mom had returned it to the animal shelter because the dog didn't bark when strangers came to the door. "What's the point of having a dog, if he's no good as a watchdog?" she said, ignoring my tears.

These small resentments and harsh words added up to me feeling a lot of anger toward my mother. Right through my teens, I longed to trade her in for someone warmer and more nurturing, like June Cleaver, Harriet Nelson and all of those other 1950s TV moms who showered kisses and kind words on their children.

I didn't realize how far my mother's Alzheimer's had progressed until three years ago, when I flew down to visit and experienced a terrible shock. My mother, always proud of her appearance and housekeeping, was dressed in dirty, disheveled clothing. She looked like a bag lady. When I asked if she wanted to comb her hair, Mom picked up her toothbrush and used that. She hadn't flushed the toilet. Her mirrors were so covered with dirt that it was impossible to see your reflection. Her kitchen cabinets and microwave were coated with food drippings. It was clear that she had no idea what food was in her refrigerator, if she had eaten, or how to use the microwave.

I tried to talk Mom into moving to New York. My dad has been dead for 15 years, and I thought she'd want to live closer to me. New York is her childhood home, too, after all. But she was – and still is – steadfast in her determination to stay in the Florida condo where she'd been so happy with my dad. At age 86, staying at home provides her with a safe haven.

I called Gil, now a doctor, and we sat down with our mother to announce that we were hiring a woman to look after her. Mom was adamant that she didn't need anyone. "I'm not a child," she said, pouting.

We hired help anyway, a saintly woman who comes each day to be sure that Mom is bathed, dressed and fed. Meanwhile, I visit when I can and call her every day.

Even now, Mom is feisty and energetic. In a strange way, she seems more joyful and alive than ever. I argue with myself about this: What does it mean to be alive? My mom, once such a go-getter that she'd attend college lectures at night, can no longer go out on her own for fear of getting lost. She sleeps long hours and at odd times, and spends many waking hours with only the television for company. Does that even count as being alive?

Yet my mom, who I once argued with every day of my life, has become a delight. She can make me laugh no matter what my mood. She spontaneously breaks into dance steps or song lyrics. If she can't remember the words to a song, she makes them up. She's a champion speller, too. I give her words to spell on the phone to help keep her mind sharp.

"You're the spelling queen of Florida!" I praise her, even as I wonder how this is possible. It takes a memory to spell. Yet, Mom has no idea what day it is or, sometimes, even who is talking with her.

Mom inspires me every day with her courage, strength and joy. She has become wise and supportive – just like those warm, loving TV mothers of my childhood. I miss her, but I also cherish every moment of this new relationship.

After I was married and had a child of my own (1987), I'd get excited whenever Mom came to visit from Florida. Then I couldn't wait until she left because all we did was argue. She'd start fights with me and say she was never coming to visit again because I was crazy. I'd tell my husband that I never wanted to see her again, but every year the same pattern repeated itself. Why? What were we getting out of it? How is it possible that I can only realize how deeply I love her now, and not then?

I am not, for one second, trying to diminish the trauma or loss of Alzheimer's, which affects over 5.5 million people in the U.S. Those numbers could skyrocket to 16 million people by 2050, and I may be among them. It's a cruel joke of a disease, robbing otherwise healthy people of their memories and their ability to care for themselves. As the disease progresses, Alzheimer's can even cause significant personality changes; many report their loved ones becoming angry or even violent. I'm so blessed that my mom is happy and content, and sounds so cheerful when I call.

"You're such a strong person, Mom," I told her recently.

I can hear the shrug in her voice. "Really?" she asked. "I always thought of myself as ordinary."

I am sad, of course, that my mother is slowly slipping away. When my brother asked me to get a copy of my parents' marriage certificate so that we could apply for VA benefits for Mom, I found myself nearly weeping in the clerk's office. My heart hurt, thinking of the vows my parents took so many years ago as young sweethearts with their lives ahead of them. Mom has no memory of this special day in her life.

What did my mother find sad or funny before? Was she happy? If she could recall only one thing in her life, the most important thing, what might it be? Getting married? Giving birth? I'll never know and she'll never remember.

Mom now struggles to remember the name of the man I've been married to for 30 years. She has signs posted around her apartment to remind her to do even the smallest daily routines: FLUSH TOILET. BRUSH TEETH. WEAR CLOTHES, TOPS AND BOTTOMS. Will her mind soon become a blank canvas?

On the other hand, why make a big deal of my mother losing her memory, when she does not? Like a child, mom lives in the moment, and most of her moments are happy ones.

Recently, she was trying to sing a song over the phone. "I made up some of the words," she confessed. "I can't remember the real ones."

"Sorry, Mom," I said. "I can't help you. I don't remember them, either. I guess we're both in trouble."

"Well, that should be the worst trouble we ever have," Mom quipped.

Our lives go by so quickly, and we don't get to pick and choose our own grand finales. We march through events that will become memories without stopping to examine them as they're happening. Then, poof! More days, months, years are behind us, gone before we know it.

"Mom, if you could wish for anything you wanted today, what would it be?"

"For my children to be healthy and happy!" she said, with such joy in her voice that I could imagine her dancing in her kitchen.

If I could wish for anything, I'd wish that Mom could grow old without any illnesses. Since I can't have that, I am grateful for this new way of being with her. If my mother hadn't gotten Alzheimer's, I would never have learned to love her so unconditionally. All of the qualities that once drove me away – her energy, her courage, her wisdom, her strength – draw me to her. I am pleased that I inherited some of her best qualities, and I'm sure that all she ever wanted was for me to be happy, healthy and fulfilled.

I am blessed that I'll be able to look back lovingly at all that my mother was as a person – and not worry about what she wasn't. To all of the daughters out there who are wishing that they had a different mother, or struggling with relationships that need healing, I hope that one day they, too, will discover that their mothers are as special as mine.

This was in 2011 and now my Diary Begins:

WHAT IS LIFE?
May 30, 2013

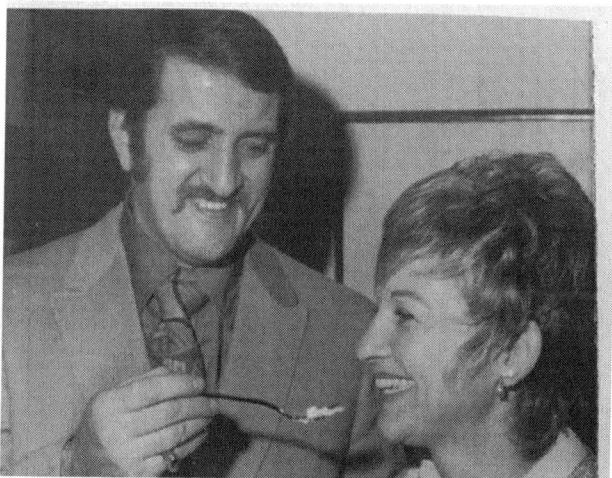

I just returned from being in Italy for two weeks, and for the first time in over eight years I had not spoken to my mother each and every day. My early morning phone calls came to a cease. Today on my first day back, I will be shortly phoning her.

Will mom know that I have not called? Will she have any realization of this? I highly doubt it, yet I can hope and dream that maybe she will say that she missed speaking to me each day.

I realize in her world that she does not know the difference. Hearing my voice and all the sentiments that I share with each phone call, hoping that I bring her joy, are all forgotten the moment our calls come to a finale. It makes me stop and wonder what the meaning of life, of being alive is.

I explain to mom why I haven't called, as if she would understand. I suppose it was my own guilt and ask her if she remembers how very much I love her. She answers that she does. I reassure her that as long as she can remember that, then that is all that matters. She quickly agrees and hopefully understands, even if it's only for the moment.

On my parent's twenty fifth anniversary, which was many moons ago, my brother and I sent them on a trip to Rome, Italy. My dad passed away eighteen years ago and mom married him at the young age of eighteen. I remembered how meaningful that trip was for my parents, and how much my mother had adored Italy.

Today, my mom has no idea of ever being in Italy, or seeing any of the treasures of the great city of Rome. It makes me wonder if this is what living is about? A life totally washed away lost out to sea as if it never existed. Her mind has become almost a blank canvas. I wonder how Alzheimer's can rob her of her life, and everything that she had once cherished.

Letter To My Mom

Mom gets to breathe the air each day and this is a miracle, one that I do not take for granted. One that I feel grateful for, yet I cannot help wondering what her life is about. She still does have some awareness, and it's the little things that I must be thankful for.

I so wish that I could have shared with her all the beauty that I saw in Italy, yet life is not always how we would like it to be. I now can only hope that for me, the memories of my trip shall remain.

My Heart Is Aching
March 15, 2013

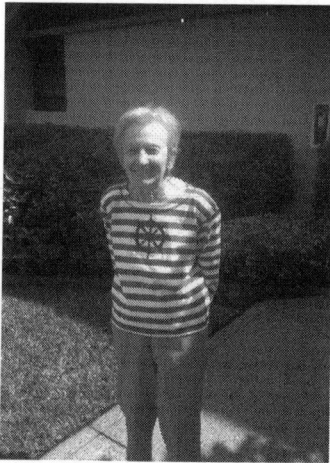

During the week I discovered that mom's money would shortly be running out. We are now getting closer to the moment, when she will have to go on Medicaid and be admitted into a nursing home. Her condition is progressing and my brother and I do not know how long she will be able to stay in her home.

As her daughter I feel saddened and am left with a heaviness I can hardly explain. I honestly feel a little lost. How can I do this to my mother? How can I abandon her? How can I just put her into a nursing home, when she still has moments of aliveness? How cruel can I be? What now are my choices?

I have so many things to think about and wish that I will be able to do the best I can for her. I do not want to upset or hurt her. The strange thing is that mom will probably not even realize what is happening, and if she does, she immediately will forget it. Her wishes and my promises to never leave her home will be broken.

My emotions are running wild. I know in my heart that I am not alone in this. I know that this is happening every day to so many other families. My writings and being able to express myself helps ease my pain.

The nursing homes are filled with so many people and have long waiting lists especially in the Alzheimer units. The beds do not free up quickly for the victims of Alzheimer's can live for years and years with this terminal illness.

I was aware that this would be happening, just not realizing when I would have to face this. Now what? Was I living in denial, or choosing to live in the moment?

Maybe we have some more time? Could mom bounce back again? Are our calculations incorrect? I think, I pray and I wonder.

I passed a homeless man several days ago and felt so troubled by seeing him. He had no place to live, no shelter, nor food to eat. It was an epiphany that hit me, for I flashed on my own mother.

Alzheimer's has stolen her life from her, yet not the love I know she can still feel. Nor the warmth and comfort of her own bed. I must stay grateful for all the blessings that we have in our life, and know that the world still has some miracles.

Aftermath:

I awoke with only thoughts of my mom. I felt queasy and I was left with frets of fears, along with all the many decisions that will have to be made. Do I bring her back to New York? Can I even find a nursing home for her? Should I have her remain in Florida, where she and my brother both live?

As I spoke to mom and shared how much I missed her, without telling her how my heart was aching, she said "do not worry, for we will get to see each other soon." My heart at that very moment broke in two.

I know that I must lighten up. Oh how I despise this horrific disease that robs you of your dignity and your life.

I cry out wanting only for my mother to hold me, as when I was a young child, and comfort me as I snuggle into her arms. I want her to reassure me, that everything will be okay.

A Long, Long Way From Home
June 21, 2013

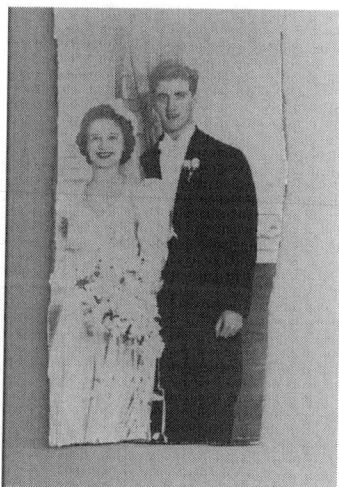

My mother and father got married on October 25th, 1942. Dad enlisted in the Navy and mom went to work on an army base in Brooklyn, N.Y. This was over seventy years ago. Unfortunately dad passed away 18 years ago and mom has no recollection of any of this.

Today my mom is not sure where her home is. When she is having a hard day she repeats many times that she wants to go home, and it is always the home that belonged to her parents. It never is the place she shared with my father, and it never is the home where she raised my brother and me.

I remember the first time after she already had Alzheimer's, that when we returned to her home after being out most of the day, she was surprised that she even lived there. I was a little in shock, since it had been her home for the last twenty something years. A home that she told me that she never wanted to leave.

My brother and I have finally made a decision that our mom must go into a nursing home. A decision that breaks my heart as it would any child who had to do this to their parent. Yet nursing homes are all filled to capacity with others' loved ones.

Since I believe Florida will be best for her, I will continue to be a long distance caregiver for mom. Another decision that unsettles me greatly. Yet as a long distance caregiver who speaks to my mother each and every day, I am filled with deep emotions like any other caregiver, no matter how close or far away they might be.

I now coordinate her care with her caregivers on a daily basis and I am in constant communication anytime an emergency seems to happen. I help plan her daily activities, her health care issues, as well as stimulating my mom by spelling, singing or simply laughing.

Am I not a caregiver? The answer is yes, just that I am a long distance caregiver. It can bother me when another caregiver thinks I may not understand because of the distance. Let me explain. I, see my mom disappearing. I also speak to her each day and go through the feelings of not being able to see her every day or once a week. I, too, am a daughter with a mom who does not know who her grandson is, nor my husband of 33 years. There are moments when she is confused about who I am, giving me the title of being "her good friend."

After I see my mom for 3-7 days in a row she has no memory that I was with her, and questions when I will be coming to visit. I do understand how horrific this disease is. It is part of my life every single moment of every single day. It does not matter how far away I may live, it is part of my life. I cannot escape any of this, nor do I want to. I am happy when she is having a good day and troubled when she is not.

The love and commitment I have for her cannot be measured. I will love and cherish every day of her life, even if she and I are a long, long way from home.

Roller Coaster Ride
July 19, 2013

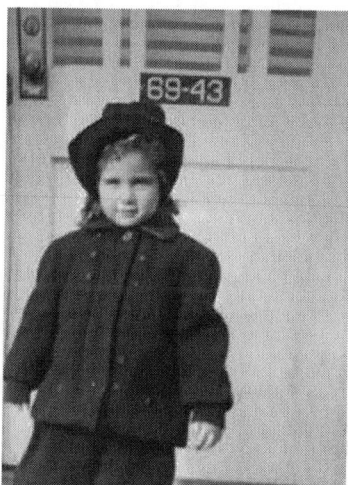

Last week was my birthday and mom had no idea of the month or day that I was born. She had no memory of giving birth to me, naming me or holding me for the very first time. She does not remember watching me grow from a child into an adult.

I feel fortunate that I can accept all of this without feeling upset. For my Birthday celebration this week I decided to have mom sing me each day the Happy Birthday song. When she arrived at "happy birthday dear ....."she blanked on my name, yet quickly replaced it with calling me "her friend", her "sweet relative" or even" her mother." I knew that I was in good company for these are all people she loved.

Since I live far away, I do not get to see her that often. My brother who visits her each week told me that she is now addressing him as her friend. She knows his name, yet usually does not remember that he is her son. Sometimes when I call she is confused thinking that she just spoke to me, when in reality she just hung up with my brother.

When I fear that she is getting worse, she somehow bounces back as if Alzheimer's is not winning. At moments there is clarity about what she is saying. Then there are the other times when she makes no sense. On these days I can hear how disconnected she is from the world.

When I do hear words flow from her they are very meaningful to me. Her being able to speak is something I never take for granted. When she insists that she does not want to spell anymore, I respect her request and just move on. I certainly do not want to frustrate her and love that she still has the ability to spell.

She makes me smile when she tells me that I should keep in touch. "Mom I call you every day." Her quick response is that her caregivers must have forgotten to tell her. After she questions where I live and I ask her where she lives, her answer is, "I live here." She has her moments of being able to answer spontaneously. She also has a knack to be able to cover up the answers that she cannot complete.

When mom calls me her friend, her relative, or her mother I still smile, yet when I hear that she is just lying in a chair staring at the ceiling, I become saddened and wonder what kind of existence does she now have?

At times her illness makes me feel like I am on a roller coaster. As she goes up and down with each elevation my heart goes along for the ride. There are the times that I stay with her and enjoy the ride, and then there are the dips that I just want to get off as quickly as I can.

Life is not always how we want it to be, yet not one day goes by that I do not feel how special it is, that I still have my mom.

WHO ARE WE?
July 26, 2013

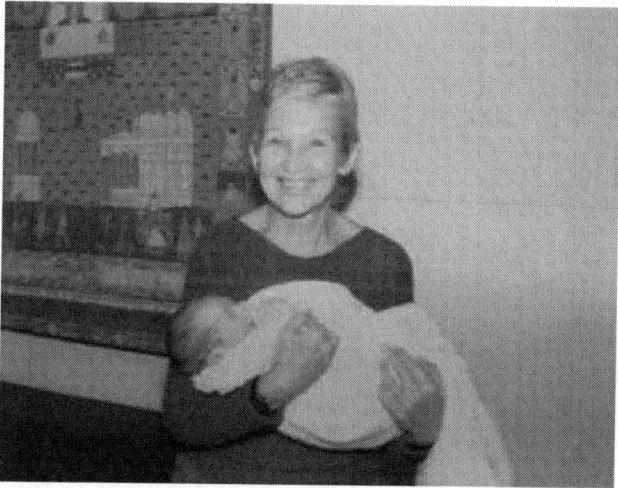

I wonder to mom who I might be this week. A mother, daughter, friend or relative? Lucky me that mom is still able to distinguish between sexes. Know need to worry that she might think I'm her son or even grandson.

In her world she can no longer explain how she sees or understands things. I sit, I listen and try to search for some clues as she sometimes shares her passing thoughts.

It amazes me how most of her life could just disappear as if in some ways it never existed.

Each day she wants to know when I will be coming to visit. She has been wanting to know this every day for the last two weeks. So much so, that I have been wondering if she realizes that I have not seen her in several months. On the opposite side of the coin, I know that if I had just visited she would not remember that either. Yet I must admit feelings of guilt have embraced me for several moments each time she mentions this.

Foolishly, I approach the topic with mom to see if she remembers what I look like and to have a little fun. "Of course I remember what you look like," she responds. "You are beautiful." "Thanks mom except you are even prettier." Ruthie says, "I am?" "Yes mom you are very pretty." With some surprise in her voice she thanks me. For in my eyes my mother was and always will be quite beautiful.

Last night I found a picture of her holding my son when he was only a few weeks old. She looked so young, and vibrant as she cuddled him. As I looked at the picture I flashed back to her life twenty five years ago. Maybe not totally perfect, yet a life filled with love, family and friends. Today mom does not know that she has a grandson. A grandson who she so adored.

Unfortunately she has macular degeneration for many years and has not been able to recognize her family in pictures. I believe that if she was able to see photos of us it could have helped her retain memories of each one of us.

Letter To My Mom

As each day goes by I wait for her to throw me my kisses. Sometimes I receive them just as I requested. Then there are the times when she just hands the phone back to her caregiver, only to be reminded that her daughter is waiting for her kisses. Other days she wonders how can she kiss me through the phone and tells me that if I want her kisses I should come over and collect them.

Either way there never is a day that I hang up without receiving her delicious kisses. Kisses that mean the world to me. Kisses that I never take for granted. Kisses that I slip into my pocket to hold close to my heart. Mom's kisses bring such warmth and mean the world to me.

On good days mom knows who I am and on off days she wonders who I am. As long as I can hear the sounds of her sweet voice it does not matter who I might be. I can only wish and pray that she may always have some memories of who we all are. For now I hold onto our brighter days never knowing when these may come to an end.

A NEVER ENDING LOVE
August 2, 2013

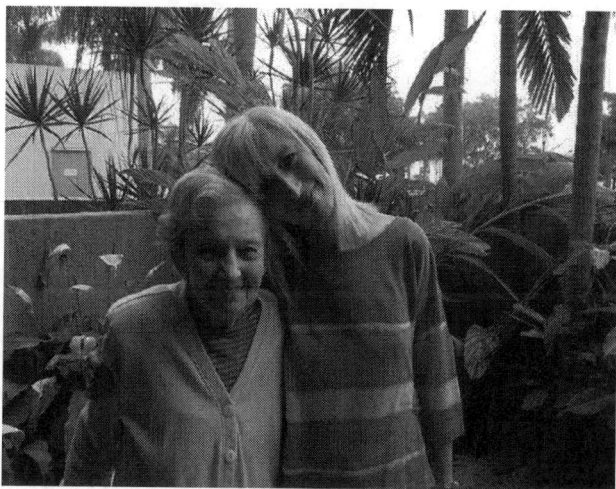

L ast week mom was having another episode with a urinary tract infection, better known as a U.T.I. It seems as if every 2 weeks the infection has been recurring. I have become a pro at recognizing the symptoms almost instantly. It's as simple as my mom mentioning that she is having some back pains along with her not wanting to end our phone calls.

At most other times she is not capable of having any lengthy conversations. Recently, she has trouble connecting her words with her thoughts. I usually can distinguish what she is trying to say, although she has trouble expressing it.

Last week, as the infection developed, we had a lengthier uplifting phone call. She was able to express all the love she felt for me and how much she missed me. As our call came to an end tears of joy fell from my eyes.

At the moment she called me her sweet, beautiful daughter my heart melted. Mom's voice sounded as gentle as she spoke these loving words. Everything seemed to connect in all the right places, as if her Alzheimer's had disappeared.

There are many things about this disease that fascinate me and with this behavior it just adds to the list. Why, when the U.T.I. starts, is mom able to continuously speak making sense and sharing past memories? She becomes animated and thrilled as she reminiscence's about these images and the thoughts that are so real to her. How can this infection affect her and have her bounce back to life?

I was overjoyed with these calls until I realized that this was the beginning of the infection. The U.T.I. would then cause her to be up all night and wander around her apartment as if she had just swallowed speed. After this for the next several days, in total exhaustion, all she wanted to do was sleep.

These conversations that once had me rejoice, now have me saying "oh no, here we go again." Unfortunately, all I am left with is a yearning for these more fulfilling moments.

The words of love that we are now able to share with one another were not always present. Life can be strange for after mom became ill, my love for her transformed into an unconditional one.

I wish that I could remove this disease from her, yet we know this is impossible. Instead, I hold onto a love for her that is never ending. A love and respect for this special lady who today has become my hero.

Update:
Mom now lives in a nursing home

THE SUN KEEPS SHINING
January 31, 2014

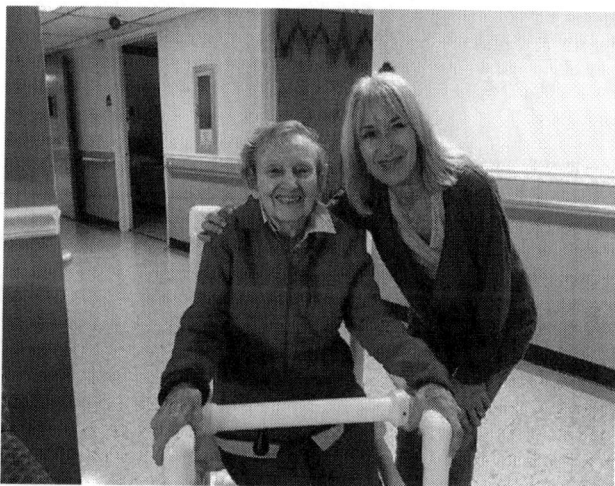

As my mother enters the latter stages of her life, whether or not she has Alzheimer's, I try to keep a smile on my face and faith in my heart. Mom will be turning ninety years old in six months. The reports from the medical team at the nursing facility tell us that she is extremely healthy.

Yet it is difficult to know how slowly or quickly her body will break down. In several ways mom is strong and appears to have much "life" left in her. Although her memory hardly exists, she still is able to communicate with everyone and stroll around in her Merry Walker. Keeping things in the correct perspective for a woman with Alzheimer's for over nine years, she is doing great.

The other evening at 8PM the nursing home phoned to tell me that mom had a large black and blue mark on her arm. I asked several questions to the nurse, "can she move her arm, is she complaining of any pain?" The nurse reassured me that everything was fine, just that she had to follow procedures to notify the family.

Thanking her for calling I hung up the phone feeling relieved yet noticed that my husband appeared to be upset. He was holding his head as if in anguish. I could not imagine what was possibly running through his mind, and only wanted to comfort him.

I was surprised by his reaction as he shared that he was fearful that was "the" phone call, telling me that my mom had passed away. At that moment tears fell from my eyes and rolled slowly down my cheeks. I knew deep in my heart that one day I will receive this call.

As I look at my mom's life, as long as she is not suffering, I can only be grateful that she is still alive. Yes I have my moments of wondering what kind of existence she has. When my mind travels down that path I quickly bring myself back to soak up the rays of sun. I know that we are not able to choose how we die, yet we get to choose how we feel and how we wish to live.

I am committed to be "in the space" of being happy. This is how my mother would want me to be. I embrace celebrating her life, her love and as of today, I will continue to allow "our" sun to keep shining through.

She's Always My Mother
February 21, 2014

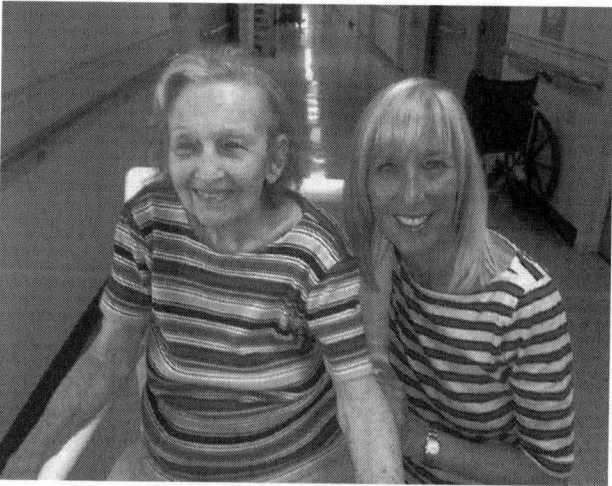

A s each day passes my mom has her moments of both distance and familiarity. It had been several days since I was able to hear her sweet voice. I phone each day and get updates from the nurses on how she is doing. I have learned to accept this, although I deeply miss the kisses that once ended all of our daily calls.

Today is what I would consider a day filled with sunshine. Mom was just walking by the nursing station as I phoned. She picked up the receiver and as I shared my sentiments with her, my eyes filled with moisture. "Mom I really miss you." She answered back in a voice that sounded free of Alzheimer's. "I miss you, too." I was thrilled to tell her that I would be visiting her in exactly four weeks. Her answer was "that's wonderful," as she dropped the phone.

It was a moment of magic for me to cherish. Somethings never change for just hearing her voice warms my heart and soul. Not one day goes by that I take for granted the miracles left of her life.

I recently watched a movie that dealt with a relationship between a mother and daughter. As it came to an end, I felt different emotions beginning to swell in me. It was the realization that I can no longer share with mom any of the meaningful things that transpire in my life.

In this respect, I recognize that this part of her has vanished. The mom who comforted me or delighted in my accomplishments is no longer capable of doing so. This awful disease has stolen this piece of her. A part that I know will never return.

Yet with it all, we still can share a deep love. What perhaps has changed is that in many ways our roles have reversed. Now it is my turn to care for her, as she had once cared for me. The truth is that no matter what my mom can or cannot do, I still am her daughter, and she will always be my mother.

Is This The Long Goodbye?
March 6, 2014

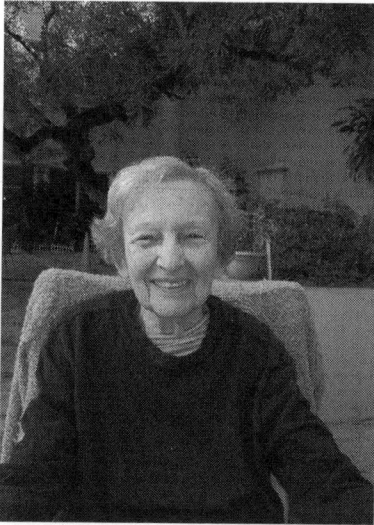

My best friend's mother just passed away after suffering from Alzheimer's for the last several years. As she sat by her mom's bed for the last week watching her fade away, I could not stop to wonder what it will be like for my mom when her time arrives. As I received the news uncontrollable tears began to run down my face. I knew a great deal of the sorrow that I was feeling was connected to my own personal grief.

At the Alzheimer support group I have been attending for almost three years, my leader has been telling me that I was in a grieving process. The first time she said this to me, I responded that I was not, because my mom, was not dying. Now I understand all, too much.

It's funny because just the other day one of mom's nurses reassured me, with delight in her voice that my mom was doing great. She shared with me how blessed my mom was and that she'll be around for quite a while. After hanging up the phone my emotions, thoughts and feelings ran rampant.

Yes, I understand that I am lucky to still have my mom, yet I also know how much more Alzheimer's can rob from her. Just thinking of how much worse she could become, as this disease progresses, leaves me feeling nauseous and sick to my stomach.

I must confess, that at moments throughout the years, knowing that there is no cure, I have wished that my mom could just close her eyes and go to sleep. I know that if she understood or could see what was happening to her, she would also wish for the same.

Today, I am in mourning for my best friend's mom and maybe also grieving for mine. For now I know that I must express what I am feeling to free myself from these haunting thoughts.

Maybe for my mother and our family this will be a long goodbye. Whatever it is I need to get back into the space of feeling grateful. In less than two weeks I will be going with my son to visit her. As long as I can see her smile and hear her say she loves me, I will push myself to come from a place of being thankful. Yet for now, I can only feel saddened.

Everlasting Love
April 4, 2014

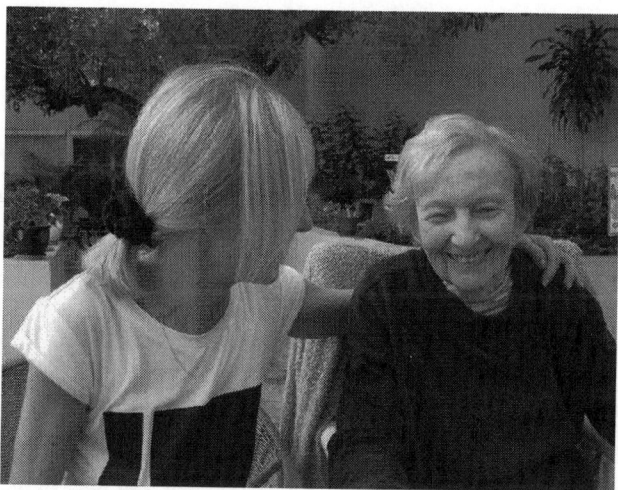

I once believed that all mothers and daughters were close. This was not necessarily true for mom and me. During my teenage years we had moved to a new town. Wanting to feel accepted by the other girls was important to me. As my newer friends came over to my home, I felt embarrassed as my mother hung around asking them many questions. My friends though didn't seem to mind, for they kept coming back.

Out of my own insecurities this left me with an uncomfortable feeling towards my mother. I know that we loved one another, just that over time it seemed that our personalities clashed more and more. While living on my own I phoned once a week, just so I wouldn't hear her complain about not hearing from me.

For many years we had our share of ups and downs. When my dad passed away, amazingly enough my mom and I got along fabulously. Then without warning our disagreements re-emerged. Yet immediately after mom became ill, there was a major shift in how I felt toward her. In a strange way I was given a second chance to love her unconditionally.

During these last months since mom entered the nursing home, I found myself filled with many different emotions. I often questioned the quality of her life. This in turn brought up feelings about my own mortality.

As her disease progresses, I have wondered if she really knows who I am. Sometimes I think yes and at other times I am not so sure. Then the other day mom described to my brother's fiancée that her daughter Lisa lived far away in New York City. Mom at that moment had some clarity. Alzheimer's disease bewilders me. How can one's whole world disappear, and then reappear only to last for a minute?

Recently I have felt some contentment. I no longer wish that mom would peacefully go to sleep. I recognize that I am blessed, for I know that I can still feel the tenderness of her touch and hear the sweetness of her voice. What I do not know is how long this will last.

While visiting I witnessed mom sharing her kisses with all the nurses. I watched and listened as she told them that she loved them. My family is fortunate that my mother is still filled with love and not frustration and anger like some others who suffer from this disease.

My mom, whom I love so deeply, has opened up my heart in many ways. This everlasting love I feel for her is embedded deep into my soul. Today and always she remains my hero.

A DEEP & PURE LOVE
April 24, 2014

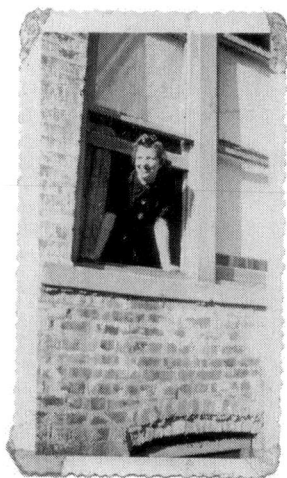

Many moons ago my mom's world was sunny and bright. It was filled with excitement, love and joy. She had no idea that one day her entire life would vanish, as if it never existed. Truth be told, neither did I, for I had never heard of Alzheimer's.

Even into her later years mom yearned to continue learning. Her passion for knowledge was important to her.

She loved to read, and taking college courses and continued to stimulate herself.

Now because of this dreadful disease almost everything she learned has disappeared. She has been robbed of memory having her entire life swept away as if it never existed.

My brother just returned to Florida after visiting me in New York. While he was here I continued to place my daily calls to the nursing home. With each call I reminded the nurses that my mother would not be having any family visitors for the next two weeks. I was aware of her being all alone and somehow I was trying to protect her. Yet in her world I'm sure she did not even realize this.

This realization had me wondering about all the other people who live in a nursing home (especially those with Alzheimer's) and have no family or friends to visit them. Perhaps they are "locked away" without any key to free them from this awful world they now live in. It is a world entwined and disguised as one.

My heart could easily break in two, if I allowed myself to think how my mom just wanders the hallways alone each day. She seems to be mesmerized, lost in her world not knowing where to go and what to do.

Although the facility that my mom now lives in has no fancy hallways, activity rooms or bedrooms, the nurses and aides all seem happy. When I think of the kindness and care that my mother is receiving I feel some sense of security and know this is what is most important.

Letter To My Mom

I realize I am fortunate that my mom is still alive. The love I feel for her is deep and pure, a bond that can never be broken. Each day I lose my mother a little more, yet each day I also get to love her some more.

Is This Life?
May 4, 2014

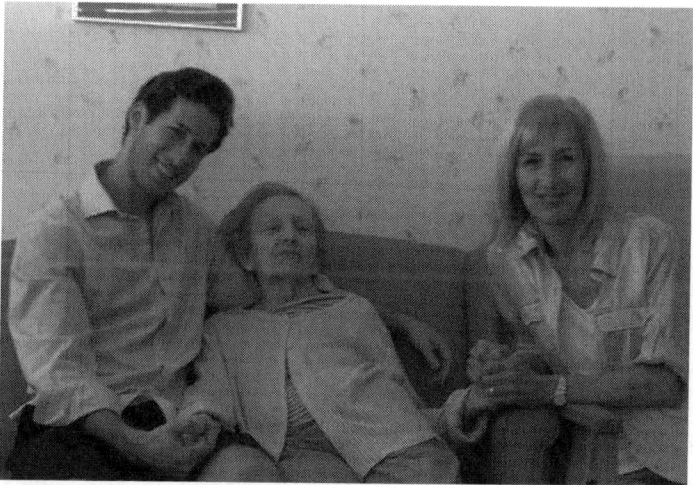

Alzheimer's is a devastating disease when compared to other illnesses for it storms in, attacks all of one's brain cells, eventually leaving nothing in its path. It deeply saddens me as I question how this is possible.

Even more frustrating is that my mom cannot describe to me what is happening to her. I can only guess what she may be thinking or feeling. Why, with most of her memory gone, does she still search everywhere for her parents? As she becomes more childlike she reverses back to her childhood.

I was fortunate to be able to speak to mom the other day which is not the usual. I shared with her by phone since I am a long distance caregiver how much I loved her and how special she was to me. She repeated the word "special" and then rambled on mixing up words so I had no clue what she was trying to say. I guess she understood what I said for one flashing moment as she quickly moved back into her own world. A world in which she lives all alone.

I often feel like a pendulum swinging back and forth with my mixed up feelings concerning her. There are times when she can make me smile and other times when I wonder what her life is all about. My heart aches thinking of her nonexistence.

I have been complimented on what a wonderful daughter I am and wish that I could truly own this. It took my mom getting dementia (ten years ago) for me to love her the way I do. Before she became ill, of course I loved her for she was my mother, yet my love and feelings for her were so different.

I regret that I was not aware of how much love for her existed inside me. Now I know how fortunate I was to be given a second chance to love her unconditionally. For this I am surely thankful.

Letter To My Mom

Since mom does not know the difference of the world she now lives in, I as her daughter, am the one who is left to feel the pain. How I wish I could rescue her from this world of no return. The destructive world of Alzheimer's.

SENTIMENTAL FEELINGS
May 15, 2014

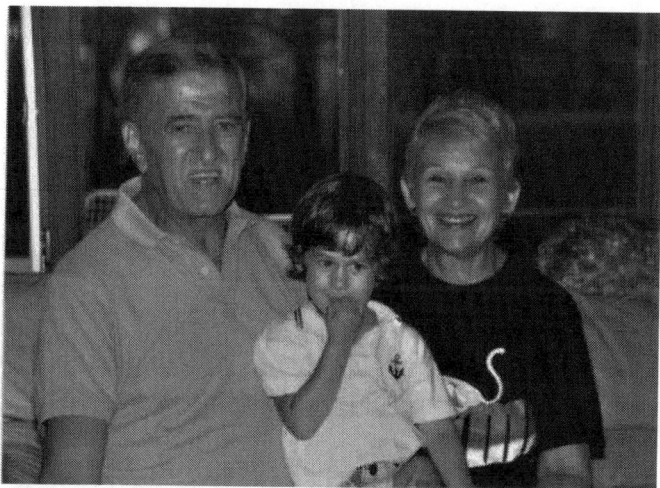

A s I write my blog post I started thinking about this past Sunday, when it was Mother's Day. Since I was able to celebrate and be with my son, mine was a special one.

Of course I missed seeing my mom and called the nursing home several times trying to wish her a Happy Mother's Day. I was unable to reach her, yet I did speak to the nurse and asked her to please send mom my love and kisses. In truth it did not really matter for mom would not understand what I was speaking about.

The distance between us keeps us apart, although I think that I was missing more the pieces of mom that are no longer present. I missed the laughter and conversations that we once shared. I missed being able to call her and describe what was happening in my life.

I wanted to get away from feeling unhappy, so I decided to choose a picture for my blog that would bring me some joy. I picked a picture of my mother and father from the mid-eighties. Logan, my son was around three years old, and mom and dad in their early sixties. These were very happy times, ones that I love to recall and reminisce about.

Today mom's journey is so different. She is slipping away more each day, and dad passed away over nineteen years ago. Life seems to go round in circles, the young grow up, and we become older, as life continues to moves on.

I choose to focus on the brighter days, ones that were filled with a love so pure and strong. I hope that the memories I have of my parents will remain with me. I want to cherish whatever life I have left, and to feel as much happiness that each day can bring.

Today is a gift for no one knows what tomorrow holds. So let's try to celebrate our lives and not hold on to the things that are troubling us.

Letter To My Mom

I wish that I could take away mom's Alzheimer's and bring her back to whole, yet I cannot. Having the strength to be thankful for what we have, is certainly a gift that I want to hold on to.

A DISTANCE FAR AWAY
June 6, 2014

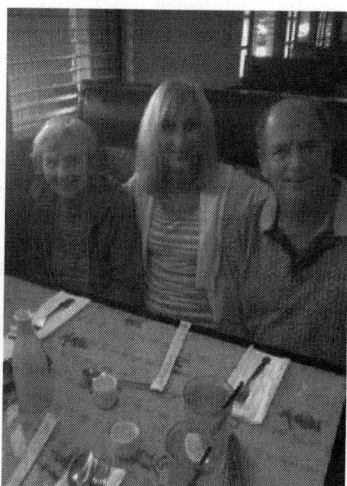

I just love her smile, laughter and the spirit that resonates throughout her. One second she can light up my life while the next moment I can feel a deep sadness within my soul for her. Living far apart does not make it any easier.

When mom first became ill and for several years there-after, I kept inviting her to move back to her home town,

New York. Her answer was always the same. "I'm never moving back, for I love my home".

I knew that it was impossible to relocate to Florida, and since my brother lived nearby, I accepted and respected her wishes. I often wondered why she would not want to be near me, nor her favorite one and only grandson. New York was where she was born and raised, a place she had lived with my father till they moved in 1985.

The distance that now lies between us is something that bothers me very much. I only get to see her every few months for a couple of days and, after I leave, she no longer knows that I was even there. I'm always left with different feelings about how she is doing. I question her mere existence of what I describe as "nothingness".

My next scheduled trip is in mid-August, when I will be celebrating mom's 90th Birthday. I'm thrilled for I have decided to make her a party at the nursing facility. A surprise one at that! Yes, she'll enjoy the cake and songs, although I wonder who this celebration really is for. Her or me?

The other morning I received a phone call from hospice who shared with excitement how well mom was doing, and that they would be removing her from their care. I replied with "oh that's good news," although that was not exactly how I was feeling.

If mom had a chance of recovery, I would be jumping for joy, yet understanding this disease, I really cannot feel too delighted.

Letter To My Mom

I wish that mom and I could be living closer. Then I would be able to spend whatever precious time I have left with her. I just know that she is a long, long way from home. A distance that is much too far away for me.

My love for her is so deep that I wish she could live another ninety years!

My Birthday Mom Cannot Remember
July 10, 2014

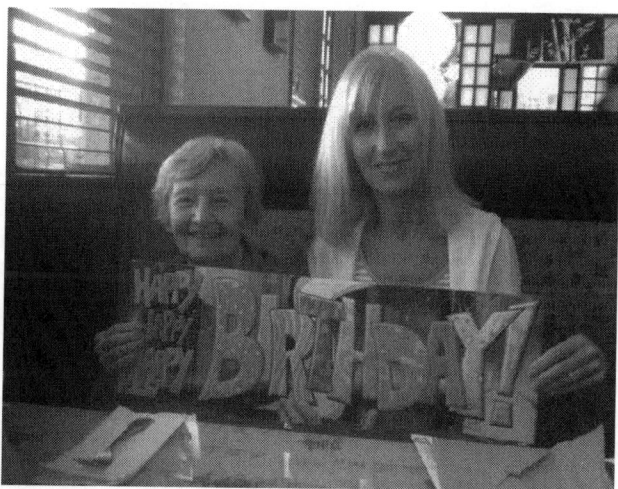

My mom gave birth to me. She raised me. She taught me right from wrong. Yet she has no idea when I was born. On good days I think she knows that I am her daughter and knows my name, and on other days she is not sure who I am. Then there are the moments that she thinks she has seven children.

After almost ten years I still find it hard to believe that Alzheimer's can rob my mother of her whole life. You would think that by now I would be able to understand this disease and how it removes one's world as if it never existed.

In my wildest imagination I cannot believe that if I were to become one of the unlucky ones, there could be a day that I, too, could no longer know my husband and son. This thought sends shock waves and chills through my entire body.

Quickly, I must remove myself from such a sad depressing thought. Today, I am free of this disease and, as I celebrate my birthday on July 12th, I will enjoy all the beautiful things that exist in my life. I will hold onto all the images that I adore and appreciate the warmth of the sun on my face. I will look at all the beauty that surrounds me and enjoy each and every day.

I cannot thank my parents enough for bringing me into this world and for all the love that they gave me. I know that if mom could find the words she would surely wish me a Happy Birthday and share with me how very much she loves me. If only she could remember.

SHE IS MY MOTHER
August 22, 2014

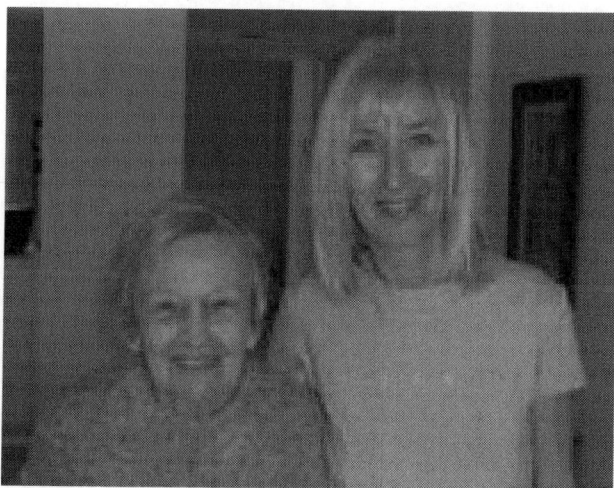

How can I find the words to express all the feelings bottled up in me since returning from spending four "precious" days with my mother? This was a special trip in which we celebrated her 90th Birthday.

The first two days mom was exuberant as she shared many different stories with us, some that made sense and others that did not. It didn't really matter what she said for it was a miracle that she was feeling so alive. Her smiles and laughter melted my heart. She was energetic and it reminded me of how she was before Alzheimer's crept into her life.

On day three she seemed more interested in running around in her Merry Walker than speaking to us, and, on day four, she expressed how tired she was, sounding more like a lost child, as she questioned every second what she should be doing.

Fortunately I was able to enjoy every moment with her and did reflect on my trip after I returned home. After sharing this with my husband I realized how much my heart ached for her and how much I already missed seeing her.

It will be four "long" months till I return to Florida. It's been difficult living so far away and having such limited time to share with her. This time in January I will be staying a whole month so I can spend more quality time with my mom.

Mom said some special things that I hope never to forget. The one I want to always remember was when we were walking down the hall together and she said that she "will always be my mother."

I know that she is my mother yet I still cannot help feeling how I want to take her in my arms and protect her from everything in her life that could possibly hurt her. I want to hold her, cuddle her, and kiss her as I tell her that everything will be alright.

Letter To My Mom

Friends and family always ask me if my mom still knows me. Yes, I want to think, yet at other times I may not be sure. Today, I believe she knows she is my mother and that I am her daughter. It's a bond that can never be broken no matter how much Alzheimer's may steal from her.

Love Does Matter
September 4, 2014

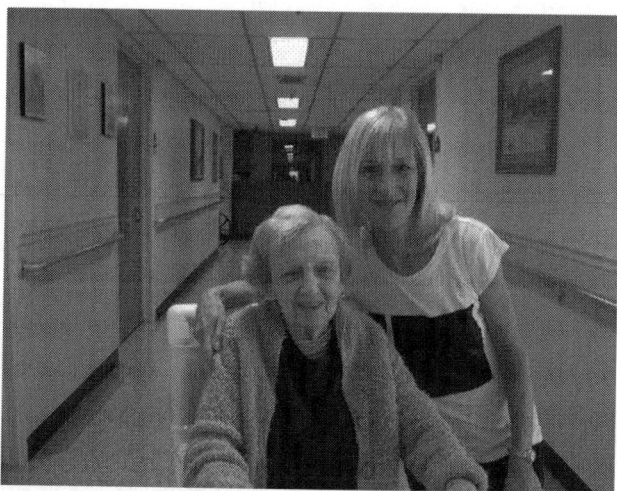

My mom has opened my heart to a world filled with love & compassion. After she became ill she blossomed into this beautiful flower with a breath of fresh air.

Although I can no longer speak to my mom every day, I awake each morning thinking of her smile and how she maneuvers around the nursing home sharing words of love.

She has become like a Buddha as she spreads joy to the aides, nurses and some of the other residents who also have Alzheimer's.

As upsetting as this disease can be it also fascinates me. I have watched as it has crept into my mother's life, removing what once existed in her universe. Now I watch as she retreats into a "new" world.

I cannot help but wonder how Alzheimer's destroys some cells quicker than others, and why some people have it for years, while others succumb to it so quickly?

What magical quality does the sound of music have to those who have this disease? I have witnessed as they come to life when they hear the melodies. I have watched when my mother interacts with those who no longer speak and I see how they look at her as they utter several words.

What makes some of their memories come to the surface while others disappear? Why does my mom think her home is with her parents? Does she go back to a time and place when she felt safe and secure? Does the world she now lives in frighten her, only wanting to return to her childhood home?

Do we think that in some ways our loved ones no longer exist and that they cannot hear our voices? Do we stop trying to communicate to them? For me, I believe they do not disappear. I believe that even when we may think so that they are still listening.

With all of this being said, then how can we deal with our loved ones who now suffer from Alzheimer's? Can we, as caregivers, understand that maybe all they want is to be loved?

This is what people with Alzheimer's have exhibited to me. They are no different than all of us for they have taught me about the power of love. They, as well as my mom, have shown me that love is all that matters.

GIVEN A SECOND CHANCE
May 28, 2015

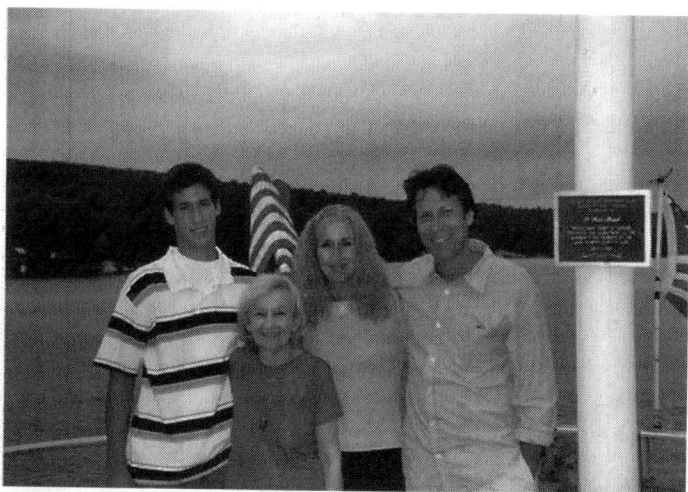

My parents were married for fifty years and dad's death was not an easy one. While he was ill and in a nursing facility for nine months, mom traveled quite a distance every day to be with him. She was strong and never complained. This was definitely a time in my life that I truly admired and respected her.

I flew down once a month to see my dad and to spend more time with mom. It was a time, as sad as it was, that I was happy to be with my mother. We were like two "teenage girls" and once again we bonded.

As I think back I can remember other times that I felt close to her, and other moments that we definitely went to battle. As I reminisce, I realize that this was the only other time, since I moved out of my childhood home, that I phoned mom every day. Not until she became ill with Alzheimer's did my daily phone calls start again. I terribly miss these calls no matter how silly some of our conversations would be. Just the sound of her voice brought warmth to my heart.

All that is left now for me is to keep calling the nursing home daily and hear the nurses tell me how mom is doing. I always say how much I miss her and request that they tell her that I love her. They reassure me that they will. I don't know why, but this makes me feel better. It makes me feel that I am connected to her.

Now that mom is further along with her disease she hardly has any memory left. For her, time stands still and yet for me it keeps moving on. Mom cannot remember the good nor the painful times. Not remembering the hurtful ones in her life, is the only blessing that goes along with having Alzheimer's.

I wish that we could be with one another as we once were. This is not possible so I like to think of her smiling face and the joy that we once were able to share. I think of the good times and all the love I have in my heart for her; leaving the tough times behind.

I might have wasted some years yet I am so thankful that I was able to get in touch with how very much I love her. I was given a second chance; one that I will never forget. This I do not take for granted.

THE GIFT OF LIFE
June 10, 2015

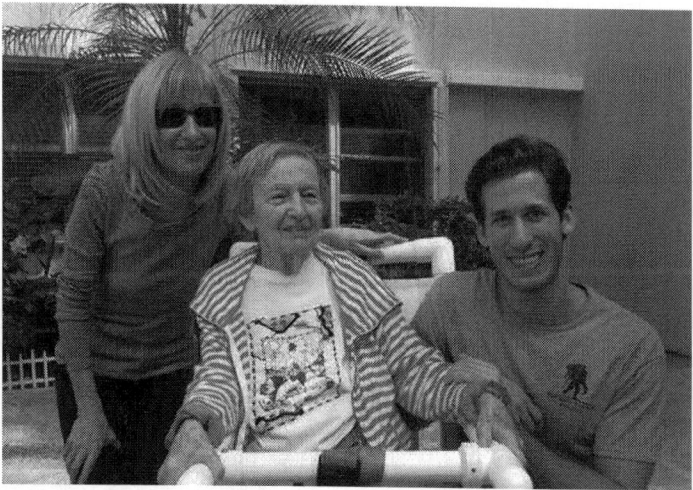

Sometimes I can forget what a gift it is to wake up each morning. Maybe I have just taken it for granted without giving it much thought. When it comes to mom, who has Alzheimer's for over twelve years, in regard to her life, my mind has traveled to many different places. There have been days when I wish that she would just go to sleep and other moments when I feel differently.

I cannot help but wonder what it is like to lose oneself and still live? I wish that mom could explain this to me. Several years ago when I presented her with a question, " Mom what is it like not to remember anything?" Her response was lovely, "although I cannot remember I know that whatever happened the day before had to be nice."

Was it possible that the mom who raised me had turned into a Buddha? Truthfully, growing up I do not remember her being so enlightened. Is it at all possible that Alzheimer's has brought out the best in her?

I wish that I could go back to my childhood and see if it was her or perhaps me acting out. Growing up is not always easy. I know that I had my share of insecurities. What could have caused me to react to her as I once did? Understanding any of this no longer matters, just being given a second chance to love her unconditionally is, undeniably, another gift.

Now all I care about is that my mom is well taken care of and "enjoying" whatever is left of her life. There is no way for me to know what she truly thinks or feels. I can only hope that when I see her smiling, singing and interacting with others that she is happy.

I have been fortunate to have recent videos of mom so whenever I feel uncertain on how she is doing, I watch them, and for those moments not only am I connected to her, I also know that she is doing great.

The gift for me is to hold onto being grateful as I watch mom "enjoy her life." I must try not to judge how her current life is, for life itself is a gift. As long as I know that she is not suffering and appears to be happy, I just want to celebrate her life, for one day it will all disappear.

MOMMY CAN YOU HEAR ME?
July 24, 2015

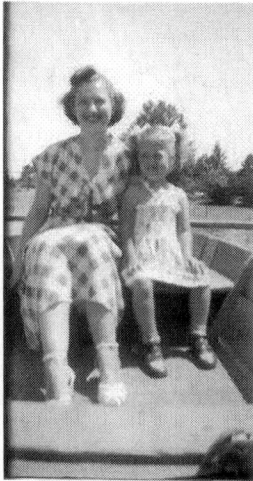

I wonder how a "grown" woman with a "grown" child can still have feelings of wanting her mother to just hold and protect her. I long to hear her say "Lisa don't worry everything will be okay. You'll see that it will all work out." Is this a feeling that perhaps will never go away, no matter how old I am?

This is an emotion that I have recently been feeling and, as each day goes by, I know that this is not possible. Yes, I am one of the "lucky "ones that my mom is still here; even if she is only half alive.

How I wish that when I tell her how much I love her she could forever remember it. Life is not always how we might like it, and I guess it's all about how we live it.

I know that these feelings will pass, yet for the last few weeks as I search my heart for answers, I cannot help wanting to be able to share them with her.

Just the other day I had my husband take me to the home that I was raised in. I lived there until I graduated college and got married. I had not driven by it in at least twenty five years. I snapped some pictures and left with sweet memories, though I realized that I no longer had a parent that I could share this with. My dad passed away over 21 years ago and my mom's Alzheimer's has taken away her memory.

Mom now travels back in time searching for her own parents. As I have suspected she has returned to a place that she, too, felt secure and loved. I'm not sure why at this time I had the burning desire to visit the setting that I grew up in.

Could it be that I am now feeling somewhat vulnerable? My son and only child in 2 months will be getting married and someday having a family of his own. Can it be the fact that life does not stand still? Am I looking at my own mortality? My husband's cousin suddenly passed away, so can this also be realizing how quickly one's life could just end?

I phoned the nursing home and started to cry with one of mom's nurses. She asked me to stop because she said that she will also start to cry. I asked a favor of her which she was happy to do. "Diane could you please go find my mother and give her a big hug for me."

Diane called me right back telling me that she found my mom and gave her a strong hug telling mom that it was from me. Mom smiled and said to the nurse, "I love you too." For the moment my tears subsided, envisioning mom doing this put a smile back on my face.

Mom's life is a part of each day of my life whether I am with her or far away. She is my mother and although life is not always as we would like it to be, our roles are now reversed. The little girl that lies deep within me is now all grown up, and although I may at times want to return there I know that it can only be in my dreams.

MOM WHOSE HAND ARE YOU HOLDING?
August 6, 2015

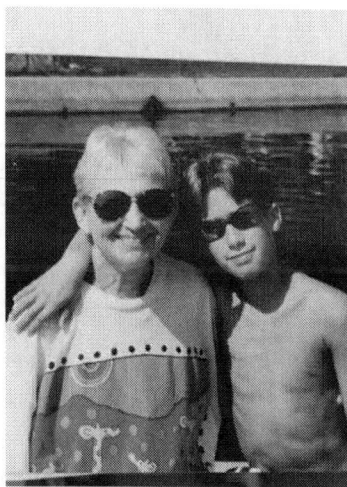

"Mom the hand you are holding is that of your one and only grandchild." I can remember all the time you spent with Logan watching his favorite TV shows and movies. It's funny how I can still hear the two of you laughing. Sometimes I'd wonder how you could sit and watch the same movie over and over again, yet that is what a loving grandmother would do for her one and only grandchild.

You no longer know who my son is nor do you understand that in six weeks he will be getting married. You met his beautiful bride-to-be in January as she came to Florida especially to meet you. "I know mom that you would be so proud of Logan, the man he has become, and would feel affection for the woman he has chosen to spend his life with."

When I think of all that you have been robbed of, I must confess it brings sadness to my heart. Alzheimer's is one of the most devastating diseases. It has the power to invade one's life and wash away a world full of memories.

Some people realize that every day is a gift and for me I hold onto each and every moment that I still can remember. I may never get Alzheimer's, yet one might say that I have a higher possibility since it runs in my family. First mom's younger brother, and then my mother.

I know that going to sleep is final and realize that I would never be able to hear your voice, see your smile or hold your hand again. I question what is better. Being alive, locked away in your own world without any knowledge of your family or existence? Yes you seem to be "happy" or should I say "content". I wonder what thoughts, if any, may cross your mind only to disappear as quickly as they come.

I believe in my heart that you would not want to be alive if you truly understood the world you now live in. For me if my world becomes like yours, I would not want to keep on living. So with much love how could I not wish for you, what I too would wish for myself.

When Logan and Julia get married at the end of September I will be thinking of you, knowing how full of happiness and pride you would have been. I promise to have you with us, if only in spirit, to celebrate this glorious occasion. I love you mom today and forever.

MOM'S NEW WORLD
October 15, 2015

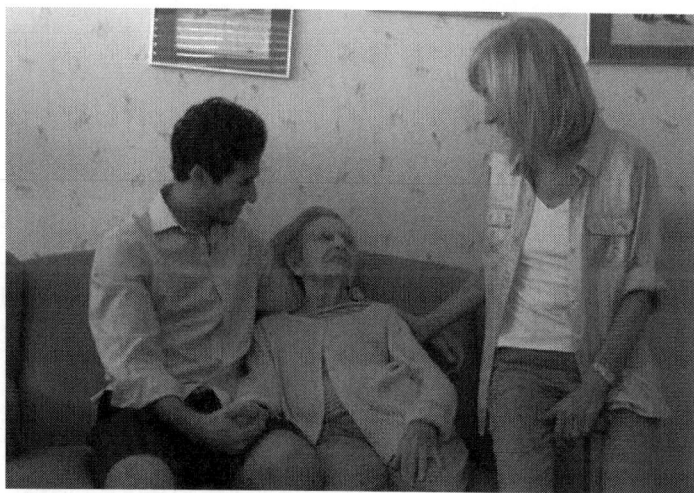

In less than three months I will be back in Florida to spend some valuable time with my mom. As the countdown begins I feel a conflict of emotions; excitement, since I will be able to see her every day, and nervousness wondering what she will be like.

When I first think of her I wonder why my feelings of love and queasiness go hand in hand. Her world seems to have stopped as if the arms of a clock were frozen in time. Why can't I just except what her "new "world now consists of?

As her daughter and caregiver I seem to envision what I would not want for her. If mom before had a looking glass, and had known what her life would have looked like, would she have asked me to "save" her from this world; a universe of Alzheimer's and a world that is still unknown?

This disease has different stages and although mom has been in stage 6 for some time now, she appears as she did a year ago. It is over twelve years since she has dementia. Is this good or bad? Is she one of the lucky ones? It is all how one looks at it. I believe that mom is not suffering so given this disease, this is all that I can ask for.

Have you ever wondered what it would be like not to know where you are, what day it is, if the sun is shining, or if it is raining? What did you eat for dinner last night and how did you spend your day? What is your favorite movie or what book did you just finish? These are the simple everyday things of life that most of us take for granted. Can you imagine not knowing any of these answers?

I question, who is the one truly suffering? Is it my mom or is it me? I think we as caregivers know that answer. Yet there is nothing we can do. I, like you, sit and wait. Fortunately I still cherish her smiles, her laughter and as each days go by, me in my world, and mom in her "new" world, I take a deep breath and keep moving on.

LIFE OF A LONG DISTANCE CAREGIVER
October 27, 2015

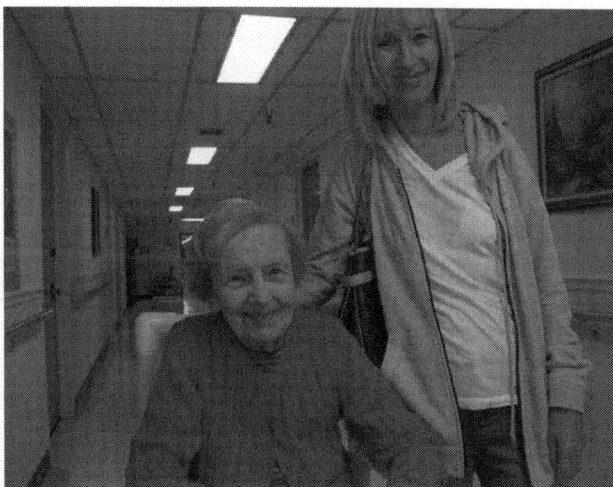

A few years ago I recall defending myself from some other caregivers. They thought I should not consider myself mom's caregiver, reasoning that since I lived far away I did not care for her in the same way that they did. Their words stung me deeply and had me momentarily question myself.

I felt compassion for their situation, yet I too, had the agony of hearing and seeing my mother disappear in front of my very eyes. One moment she knew my name and the next she had no idea who I was. My heart felt equally broken as theirs and I questioned why would they judge me?

Was I any less of a daughter to my mother because I did not live near her? Unfortunately, I could not just pick up and move to another state, and my mother refused to leave her home. I am my mother's daughter which will never change no matter how many miles may separate us.

For years, before moving mom into the nursing home, I spoke to her caregivers every single day to hear how she was doing and to help plan her day. I questioned what she ate, if she took her vitamins and if she gave them a hard time when she was being bathed. I also delighted in hearing how mom loved to sing along to the CD'S that I made for.

There were moments when mom sounded great and there were other times when I was so frightened yet unable to just jump in my car and rush over to her. I remember when they called an ambulance to take mom to the emergency room after her aides discovered she had bruises (from a fall) that she could not tell us about. Then there were the times she was hallucinating which was due to a urinary tract infection (UTI).

Once, when she was in the rehab hospital I spoke to the physical therapist who told me that my mother was not following instructions. I responded "how could mom possibly remember what you just said since she has Alzheimer's." The therapist answered, "Oh I didn't know she had dementia."

Then there was the time I received a call from a first response team who was not able to reach my brother. Mom's neighbors reported her "just sitting" outside her apartment on the curb. Her caregiver left for the day and because of confusion mom went to sit outside to wait for her. You would think that one of her neighbors would have just brought her back into her home. After all these years of knowing her how could they now just shun her like this?

The time was approaching to place mom into a nursing home, my brother and I realizing she needed twenty-four hour care. Talk about feeling guilty and confused. How could we do this to mom? Her wishes were to stay in her home till she died.

Mom now has been in a nursing home for 3 ½ years and my brother and I know that it was the correct thing to do. I still call every day and speak to the nurses to see how she is doing. I may only get to visit her every few months yet the staff knows that I take a very active interest in her well-being. Mom no longer knows where she is living yet my brother and I feel secure with the care that she is receiving.

So with deep thought my question is: am I any less of a daughter than the others since I am a long distance caregiver? The answer is clear to me. I am my mother's daughter and no matter how many miles apart we are the love and concern I have for her is as deep as the bottom of the ocean. She is my mother and I will always be her daughter, which also includes being her caregiver.

ALZHEIMER'S COULD THERE BE A SILVER LINING?
March 3, 2016

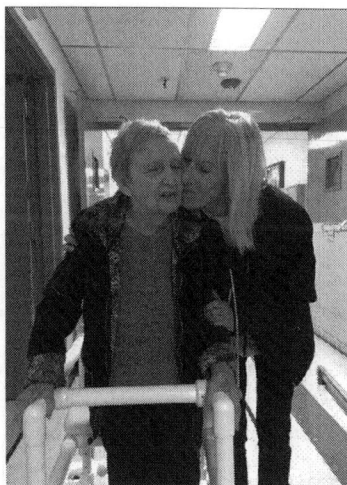

In that my mother lives in Florida and I reside in New York, it had been a while since my husband and I had visited her. What made this trip extra special was the fact that we would be seeing her every day for an entire month. This was not one of my usual quick three day visits. It was one we did the year before and both of us knew how meaningful and rewarding it would be.

Upon arriving at the nursing home I nervously asked my husband to sign in as we proceeded to the second floor. Although many of the patients on this floor have Alzheimer's it is not a locked unit. Fortunately for us mom has never been one of the wanderers. She has never been on any medication for agitation, depression or any other ailments. Except for Alzheimer's and macular degeneration, at the age of 91, she is in "perfect" health.

As I exited from the elevator I quickly hurried to the nurse's station to introduce myself to a new nurse whom I never met, and to find out where my mom was. Was she walking around the second floor in her Merry Walker or was she still in bed? I was told that she was "off and running." I circled the floor and found mom in a corridor all alone. As I observed her I noticed that she was walking much slower. The good news was that she was still mobile.

I went to her and softly kissed her cheek as my eyes filled with tears. Mom was happy to see "someone" yet she had no idea that I was her daughter. It appeared that she was slipping further into the disease. The first thing she said to me after I kissed her was "kill me." I asked her what she said as she quickly corrected herself and said "kiss me." I wondered if this was a Freudian slip, did she actually say it in a moment of clarity, or was this something that she might have really wished for?

On day two mom, as soon as she saw us, said that she was very tired yet that she also felt happy. Was there some recollection to who I was? Was it the sound of my voice, my touch of her skin, or were my kisses different than the ones she receives from the nurses and aides?

As we went into a sitting room that we nicknamed "the living room" we took mom out of her chair and sat down together on a couch. Mom held onto my hand and squeezed tightly, as if she never wanted to let go. The way she kept smiling at me made me believe that she was aware that I was her daughter.

We played some songs from You Tube that I knew she was once familiar with. She became alive as she sang along to Frank Sinatra's "My Way" and "New York, New York". It never stops to amaze me how much music cheers the soul of those who suffer from this disease. It is the best "healing" medication there is. The magic of music somehow opens up their world; a world that no longer exits.

The following day mom refused to get out of bed. We found her laying still in a fetal position. She hardly spoke and refused to get up. I once again held her hand and was surprised and a little relieved when she threw me a kiss and told me that she loved me. It was a difficult visit just seeing her trapped and lost in her own world.

Unfortunately mom cannot describe or tell us what might be bothering her. Maybe she didn't sleep last night or maybe she was not feeling well.

On day four I was feeling anxious and filled with antici-
pation on how we would find her. It turned out to be a day
filled with miracles. Mom was up and about in her Merry
Walker. As we approached her she told us that she was
looking all over for us. We went to "hang out" in the living
room and seeing how lucid mom was, I asked her to spell
some words. This was something that she once did well.
We ambitiously asked her to spell orange, purple, yellow,
sunshine, apple, and with amazement, she quickly spelt
each word correctly.

This disease remains such a mystery to me. After thirteen years I am still baffled after witnessing things with
mom's mind. Since entering the nursing home why does
she run around searching for her parents? She speaks
about them in such present tense and only wants to go
home believing that they are worried and waiting for her.
She repeats this same scenario almost every day.

I wonder how she can still spell when spelling takes
a memory and how hearing music bring back the words
that have long been forgotten? How can she be lucid one
moment, then disappear into her world the next?

Yes, Alzheimer's is one of the cruelest disease's that
eventually takes your life. Some people live with it for
years and others succumb rather quickly. My mom has
Alzheimer's for many years and if there could be any sil-
ver lining then I have found one. Mom cannot remember
anything in her life that caused her any pain or suffering.
She does not really understand what has happened to her,
and if she does the thought passes through her brain so

quickly that she can "peacefully" go back into the world she now lives in.

As her daughter first, and her caregiver second, I believe that I am the one that feels her pain; yet I too have been so fortunate to have been able to live in the world of being thankful & grateful for whatever mom and I still can share.

THE SUN WAS TRULY SHINING
March 14, 2016

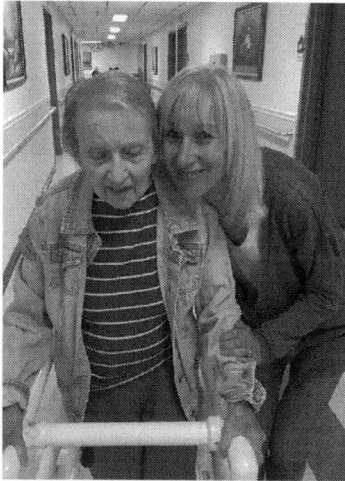

As the first week of our visit came to an end, I was hoping that mom would become more aware. Fortunately, during week one, each day mom became a little more alive. I could see she was yearning for the warmth of our human touch. I only wished that she would recognize me as her daughter. Alzheimer's disease has stolen from mom not only her identity, but also those whom she loved.

Since our arrival, each day was either cloudy or raining with only hints of sun peeking through. The weather was not cooperating although this was not why we came to Florida. It was to spend some quality time for the entire month with mom.

As week two began I awoke to the first day the sun was shining. There was not one single cloud in the sky. It was a crystal clear day and I felt the warmth from its rays, yet I could also not help but feel a pang in my heart. My heart ached and I knew it was somehow connected to mom and the sunshine. I wondered how I could feel so sad on such a sunny day. I soon realized the heaviness I felt was that I could not share this day with her. I knew she was probably incapable of enjoying it.

Truthfully speaking she has no awareness of what is happening in "our" world. She cannot recognize whether the sky is cloudy or filled with brilliant sunshine. She does not care and perhaps the world she now lives in could be described as a "safe haven".

I wished that I could have taken her out to feel the warmth of the white sand as we strolled on the beach. I wanted mom to be able to put her toes in the sparkling water and feel the suns reflection on her body. This was a pastime that we once shared, one that I knew she loved. I was feeling sad just knowing she was missing out on this glorious day.

As my husband and I approached the nursing home I realized that I had to quickly shake off these negative thoughts and feelings that were embedded in my soul.

Letter To My Mom

As we approached mom, her first words were "I'm too young to die." She then tenderly touched my hand and kept repeating "stay with me," as we circled the hallways of the facility. I wondered what she could possibly be thinking.

On the tenth day my cousin's family came to visit mom. Mom had seven visitors all at once. I was hoping that all the noise and attention would not disturb her. Sometimes the sound of noise can be disorienting for those who suffer from Alzheimer's. I know that mom had no idea who anyone was, yet the mere fact that my cousin came and with her family meant the world to me.

The following day I was pretty certain we would find mom curled up in bed feeling exhausted. Instead we found her walking around in her Merry Walker filled with energy, beaming with happiness. She immediately asked my husband if he would be her "boyfriend" quickly adding that she was only kidding. For that moment mom was back, quick witted and sharp as she could be.

As the day came to an end, this visit with mom is one that I hope never to forget. It became a day when that the sun was truly shining!

Is This A Life Worth Living?
April 6, 2016

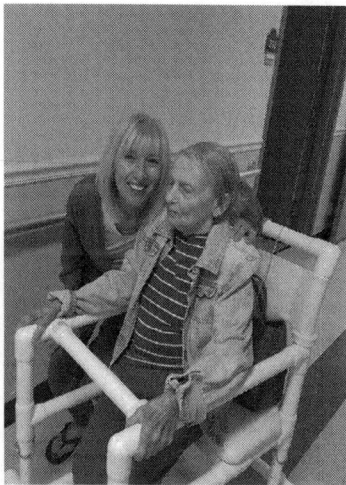

As my month long visit comes to an end my daily trips to see mom get harder and harder. I can feel my emotions surfacing, taking over as if I were riding a roller coaster.

I awake each morning feeling like I could cry. I feel the pain of leaving her. In some ways I think I am deserting her. How I wish that I lived near mom so I could cuddle and care for her. I have this burning desire to protect her, as if she were my own child.

In many ways our roles have reversed, yet I yearn to hear her call my name. Even if it is for a brief moment I want her to know that I am her daughter.

Saying goodbye never gets easier. It's not just leaving a parent, but also not knowing how much more of her will be left when I return.

I wonder if mom could have a sixth sense for on one of the final days of my visit my husband and I found her in bed. We caught her having a dream as she was having a lengthy conversation with someone. After she awoke she continued speaking to us with phrases that had a "philosophical" meaning. She shared her feelings on how we should appreciate our life and be kind to one another.

Could mom possibly know what I was feeling these last few days, or could this have been a miracle from above? Did she want to send me back to New York feeling complete? I felt like she was a Buddhist or an angel who just spread her wings.

I realize that life is not fair. Some people die young and some live to an old ripe age. Some people in their nineties are still driving their cars while others have moved into nursing homes unable to care for themselves. None of us know what lies ahead and for this we need to be grateful for each day that we are alive.

Mom lives a life I hope never to endure for myself or any of my other loved ones. Her life was once so full and now she is locked away in her own universe. It is hard to explain yet sometimes it appears that she is trapped in the unknown world of the "Twilight Zone".

Who am I to really judge if this is a life worth living. I wish that I could wave a magic wand and bring her back into the real world.

I only wish that mom could understand all the love I have for her. I am fortunate to have been given a second chance to love her in a way that I never before realized. Mom has become my hero. Her strength and courage inspires me each and every day.

THE POWER OF TOUCH
April 19, 2016

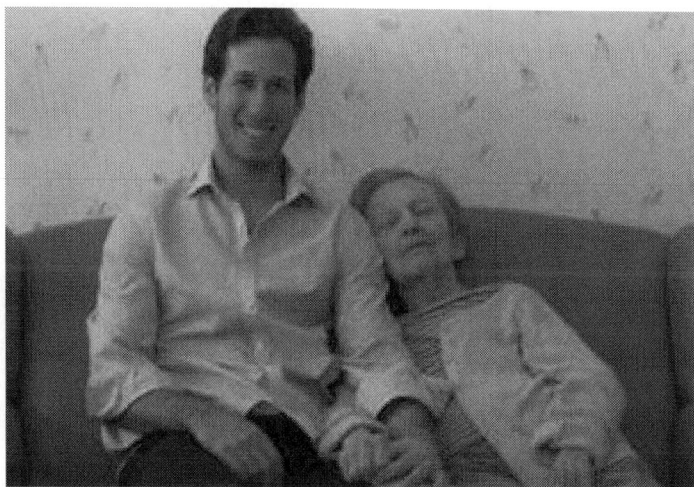

I have read that physical touch is one of five ways people communicate and receive emotional love. It is also stated just reaching out and taking someone's hand can be the beginning of a journey. For me holding hands was the tenderness moments that my mother and I shared during my month long visit.

As we held each other's hands our fingers intertwined like never before. It felt to me as if I never wanted to let go. It was at that very second that I became aware of how meaningful human touch was with my mother. Mom's fingers spoke words to me. They told me how much she loved me as I felt her warmth and tenderness like never before.

Every once in a while she'd open her eyes, look at me, squeeze my hand and smile. How I yearned to know what she was thinking, although on this day most of her words remained silent. Suffering for thirteen years this disease has been removing her use of language.

On this particular day as I played some of mom's favorite music she held my hand tightly as she either hummed along or softly spoke a few words to let me know how beautiful the music was. Heavens doors seemed to open as we listened to Susan Boyles sing "I Dreamed A Dream", Andre Bocelli and Pachelbel Canon in D major.

We held each other's hands for hours as if we were young lovers. Yet this was different, it was my mother that I was touching. We needed no words, just holding hands said it all. We both held on so affectionately as if never wanting to let go. Each day thereafter I hungered for my mother's touch, meaning more to me than I could have ever imagined.

I am now back in New York while mom remains in Florida. Not only do I miss her deeply I very much miss the caressing of our hands. I miss her touch, her warmth her tenderness which filled my heart with love.

What does the human touch mean to you? Is it feeling the warmth and caring of another human being? Or is it perhaps feeling loved? Is it embracing another person?

Whatever it means to you, for me, it was intimate. So different than one that I could have ever dreamed that I would be able to share with my mother. It is for me a love that has come full circle and now is complete.

How Is Mom Doing?
April 27, 2016

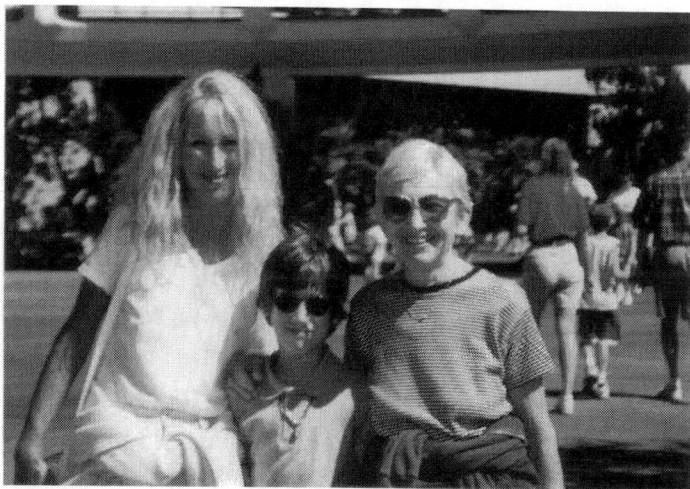

My dad passed away 22 years ago and my son Logan is now 28 years old. For the last three years mom has been living in a nursing home. She has dementia and macular degeneration, takes no medication and is in perfect health.

In many ways my family has much to celebrate and be thankful for. Occasionally friends will ask this one question of me. "How is your mom doing?" I often answer, "My mom is doing good considering that she's had Alzheimer's for the last 13 years."

Several weeks ago I stopped to really think about this question. I thought about mom, a lady who has no idea about the life she once lived.

She no longer understands that she needs to get dressed each day, brush her teeth, or comb her hair.

She never thinks about what she'd like to eat, or what restaurant she'd like to go to.

She has no idea what has transpired in the world or that we just celebrated Thanksgiving.

She has no fear of Ebola or terrorism.

She does not understand that her only grandchild just got married. In fact, she does not really remember that she has a grandchild.

She no longer needs to think about what friend she might like to spend the day with, or what movie she would like to go see.

She no longer has to make any decisions on whether she'd like to take a walk in the park, stroll on the beach, or go to her favorite museum.

She does not remember that she was married for 50 years. She does not remember giving birth to her two children.

Letter To My Mom

She never has to decide where she'd like to go on vacation or what country she'd like to travel to. Life for her has certainly become "carefree".

Mom has no understanding of how her life has been wiped away by such a horrific disease. So how is my mom doing? She'd doing well, and how am I doing? I'm also doing well, which is a conscious decision I have made.

Today there is no cure for Alzheimer's. So as long as I believe that my mom is "happy" and not in any pain the only thing left for me to do is to love her completely.

My Mom I Love Her So
August 3, 2016

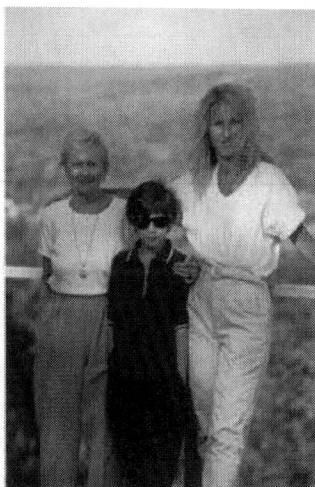

One evening, several weeks ago, I received a call from the nursing home. One can imagine the uncertainty I felt when I answered the phone.

Immediately the nurse said "everything's okay I just need to tell you that your mom was unresponsive today." As I heard the word "unresponsive" my heart sank. I asked many questions as she proceeded to explain what had transpired.

My husband said as he looked at me that I appeared to have lost all the color in my face. His first thought was that mom had passed away until he heard me repeating what the nurse was saying.

I did not sleep soundly that night fearful that I would get a call that mom had passed away. The next morning my brother rushed to the nursing home where tests were already being performed.

Mom's unresponsiveness only lasted for a few moments, yet it was something that was new and felt quite scary. The blood results found that mom (93 years in August), in several ways resembled a 40 year old. Her constitution is amazing.

The next day I booked a plane to go and see her. Before leaving I called several times each day to make sure that she was doing okay. Each time I was told that she was running around in her Merry Walker. Mom bounced back rather quickly and I was happy that I was going to see her, even if it was just for three days.

After returning home my body felt stressed and my heart ached as if I was going through withdrawal. I missed seeing her and could not stop thinking about her. Again I kept phoning the nursing home to see how she was doing. Mom was doing fine, it was me who needed to "mend".

I kept thinking is she looking for me? Does she wonder where I am? Is she missing holding my hand, singing songs, or our silly conversations? Does she yearn to see me like a teenage girl, or am I in this all by myself? Is my heart hurting alone or can she also feel the pain?

I write as if she is my lover. No, she's my mother, yet I love her in so many similar ways. I know the answers to all these questions for the second I am no longer in her sight, she does not know that I was even there. In fact, when I am with her, she does not always know that I am her daughter.

None of this matters for in my heart I deeply believe that in hers, we share a bond that only a mother and daughter could feel.

WHAT'S IT ALL ABOUT?...ALFIE
August 21, 2016

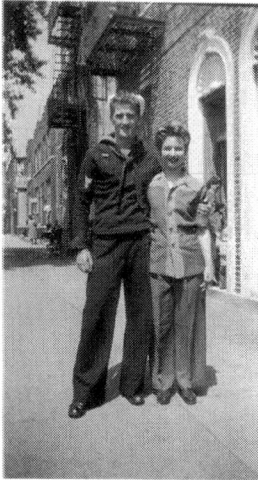

I cannot get out of my head the song Alfie; "What's it all about Alfie? Is it just for the moment we live?"

In the world mom lives in, each day, after she wakes up her aides need to take extensive care of her. After she is washed and dressed she is then placed in her Merry Walker where she spends hours walking the halls of the nursing home in search of something or someone.

How I wish I could know who is that something or someone she is searching for. Is it her parents, or could it be me? Probably her mom and dad since she frequently is talking and looking for them.

As I sit and ponder what really exists in my mother's mind I wonder who she thinks she is. Unfortunately, mom can no longer provide me the answers I yearn to hear.

How I hunger to ask her; are you happy or are you sad? Are you frightened or are you okay? Are you lonely? Is there anything that you would like me to do for you? Is there something that you would like to tell me? Do you know what is happening to you? Can you understand how deeply I love you?

I know there is a universe that mom now lives in, one that is real to her. Yet for me I cannot help but wonder what is going on in her world. So as the song goes "What's it all about Alfie? Is it just for the moment we live?"

I realize there are things that I will never understand and questions that will never be answered, yet as her daughter I need to believe that in her world she is sound, safe and happy.

After all these years, as each day goes by, Alzheimer's still remains a mystery to all of us. I have read much about Amyloid plaques and tangles, yet the scientists are unable to understand what is really going on in the minds of people with Alzheimer's.

Now, all I can do is hope and pray that one day they will find a cure or even a prevention for this horrific disease.

What Comes First Daughter or Caregiver?
October 27, 2016

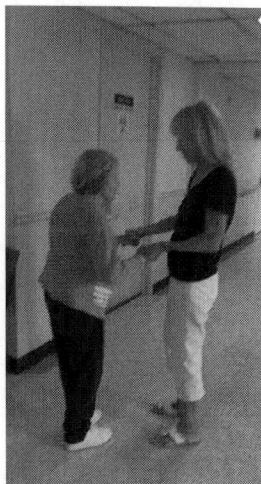

When I am interviewed for a podcast or radio show I feel a pain when I am introduced as my mother's caregiver; for in my very soul, deep in my heart, I am first my mother's daughter and then her caregiver.

After looking up both words in the dictionary I found several different meanings. A daughter is a female child or person in relation to parents; a caregiver is a person who cares for someone who is sick or disabled.

A name I wish to be called is mom's "care-daughter". Although "care-daughter" does not exist in the dictionary I truly prefer the way it sounds.

In the last several years I know our roles have reversed, although what remains is that I am her daughter.

Recently, I shared with a friend that on my last visit with mom it was so meaningful to just hold her hand. Since my return my friend asked, did I miss holding my mother's hand? My answer was simple. "No I don't miss holding her hand, what I do miss is not being able to share my life with her. Mom is still alive yet the world she now lives in is a world I do not exist in."

I then reversed the question and asked "can you ever imagine one day not knowing that you have two children named Billy and Alice, or that you are married for forty years, or that you have two sisters?" She looked at me and could not answer.

I have come to realize that unless you have a loved one with Alzheimer's you cannot really understand this disease.

Since mom is living with this disease for over fourteen years I know how fortunate I have been to still have this time to spend with her, yet throughout the years, I have begun saying my "goodbyes".

Letter To My Mom

Alzheimer's disease is not only mind boggling, it also can be a very long journey as we watch our loved ones disappear. They no longer live in our world so we somehow must learn to live in theirs.

Regardless of how many years mom and I may have left, today and always, she is my mother, and I will first always be her daughter. I love you mom, more than words could ever say.

THE WORLD SHE NOW LIVES IN
December 23, 2016

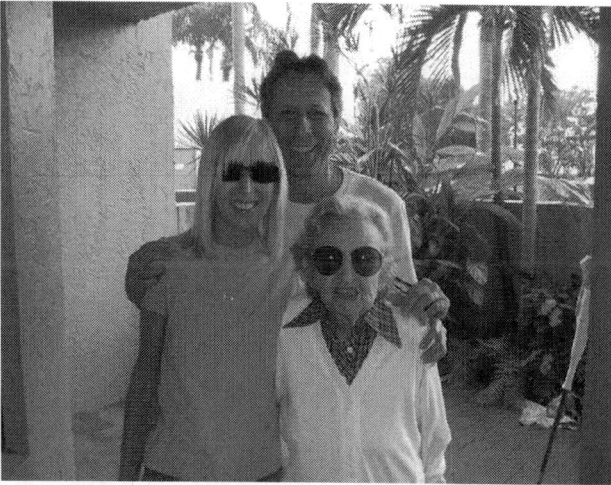

In a few days I will be arriving in Florida to see my mother. I did this for the last three years, allowing me to spend an entire month with her. I usually feel a combination of excitement and nervousness, yet this year I am scared.

My brother recently sent me a video which troubled me. Mom seemed far more advanced almost as if she did not exist. She mumbled a few words, was unresponsive, not having much expression. I am hoping with my daily visits she will somehow reappear.

This past Friday night I knew all too well that she had no idea of the day, time or year. She is unaware that I will soon be coming to see her. She most likely has no idea that I even exist. The world that is so present in my universe does not exist in hers.

Alzheimer's has taken over. It has conquered and left mom with little awareness of any life on this planet. She is locked away in a land of make believe, a land of no existence. Gracefully she appears not to be suffering.

This journey that we are now on is getting much more difficult. I am filled with guilt and sadness, at moments wanting her to go to sleep. How could I wish for this with my own mother? Am I cruel? Am I inhumane?

While she is still alive she rarely ever smiles. When someone with Alzheimer's does not smile, and shows little emotion, it appears that they are nearing the end. In mom's case given her constitution, the end may not be so near.

I miss her deeply and being able to touch her face and hold her hand should be enough. How I yearn to share my life with her wishing that she could understand when I whisper the words "I love you".

Alzheimer's is a cruel disease that wipes away ones dignity and life as it enters and attacks their brain cells.

Letter To My Mom

Some people succumb rather quickly, while my mother has Alzheimer's for fourteen years and still counting.

At this moment many scientists are searching for a prevention or cure and are hoping that within 15- 20 years it will come. That is a long time away but for future generations it would be a blessing.

Love, Love, Love
December 28, 2016

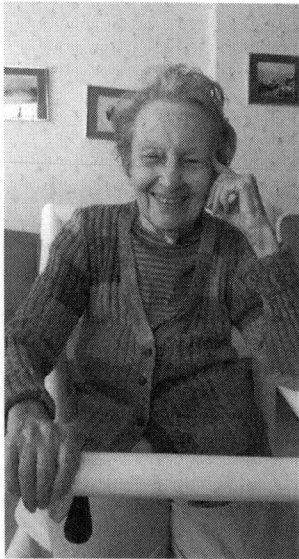

My brother called me the other day while he was visiting our mother at the nursing home. I unfortunately missed the call yet he left a message asking mom to say hello to me. Hearing her say "Hi Lisa," immediately brought me back to a time when mom was whole. Her voice was filled with strength and definition.

Mom sounded free and clear of Alzheimer's. Her voice and tone was that of the mom I always knew. I wondered how this could be. Is it possible that mom still has moments of being herself? At these times could she have a flashing thought wondering what is happening to her? A thought that disappears as quickly as it comes.

I will never know the answers and maybe its better that way. I desire only to protect her from anything that can cause her heartache or pain. I wish to cuddle her in my arms as if she were my own child and reassure her that everything will be okay.

I realize that whatever is left with mom is to try to enjoy the moments we have together. I want to sit with her, talk to her, touch her and hold her. I want to sing with her, laugh with her and just be there for her. I want to show her, and have her feel, all the love I have for her; never questioning whether she knows if I am her daughter.

There are things that we can never get back yet I want to remember the things that I loved, and also the things she did that drove me crazy. I want to remember her lectures to me, her humor, her support and all her imperfections. She was never perfect yet neither was I.

She is still my mom, and the journey that we have been on together for over fourteen years has at times been difficult yet also one filled with love.

Letter To My Mom

I cannot take Alzheimer's from her and though it breaks my heart as I watch her disappear, it has opened my heart to a place that I did not realize even existed. It has made me closer with her and has turned my love into one that is unconditional.

THE FINAL CHAPTER
March 5, 2017

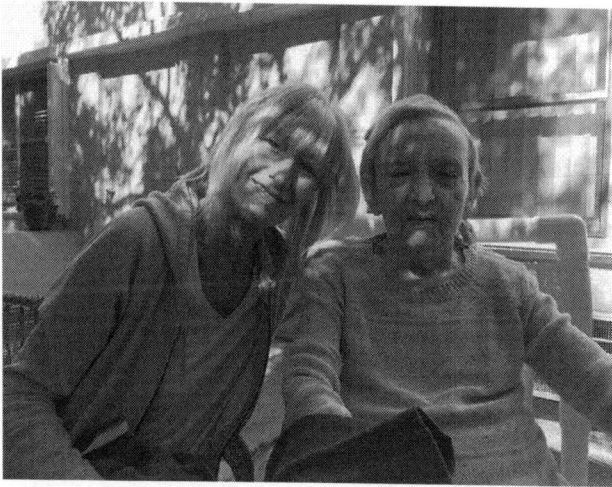

For the last fourteen years I have witnessed my mother slowly disappearing from Alzheimer's. With a heavy heart I go through the process of grieving and realize that through my writings I have begun to heal myself.

Is it possible for me to share all the feelings that are so deeply embedded within my soul?

This past January my husband and I were in Florida to spend each day with her. In the past four years, each January, we witnessed mom transform day by day as she became more aware of the world around her.

I had realized that mom would not be like last year, yet I could never have imagined that from a bad cold her world and mine would shatter.

I mainly sat by her side, held her hand, stroked her face and told her how much I loved her. Mom has now entered into in the last stages of Alzheimer's. How I wish that I could have her peacefully go to sleep; instead of what could take many months or years for her to say goodbye.

Her words are now seldom, her eyes mostly shut closed. Her walking around the nursing home has come to a halt for she no longer has the will nor energy to carry on.

She occasionally opens her eyes and, once in a while, she would smile. I was able to steal a few kisses yet even the sound of music that once delighted her, could not bring forth any signs of joy.

Witnessing her withdraw from the world was quite painful. As my thoughts surfaced I took to pen and paper to share my most inner deep feelings. My prayers were not answered as I had prayed for her to pass away. I knew that mom would never want to exist like this. I also wanted to take away the pain I was feeling, knowing that there could be no recovery.

Letter To My Mom

I question why my mom got sick while I was here? Why couldn't we have been able to share some special moments like we had done in previous years? Couldn't she have waited to after I left? How silly of me to even think this way. No one gets to choose when or where.

Whirlwind of A Ride
March 27, 2017

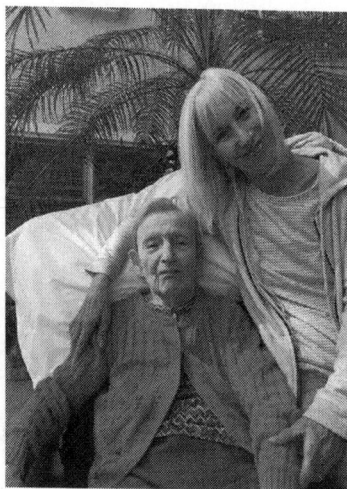

Since mom became quite ill during my visit in January I have been affected in many way. Just watching her disappear from Alzheimer's for the last fourteen years had been grueling enough. I had to accept that her world was climaxing and could end rather quickly.

Even though I have prepared myself, I realize that when the time comes I will be in mourning for the loss of my mother. She will become just another statistic and I will be parentless like so many others my age.

People often ask if I fear that I will get Alzheimer's. My answer is always the same. I do not fear it, and I am aware, when I cannot remember something as simple as an actor's name. Not only does my mother have Alzheimer's her younger brother also had it and passed away after just a few years. I recognize that my chances are greater than someone else whose family has no history of this disease.

Recently mom's "world", if only for the moment has "improved "in a way that I was not ready for. Maybe I didn't really wish for this to happen. She seems to have bounced back with a reborn energy. Her nurse reassured me that mom was once again back to "herself", feisty, eating well and maybe even better than before. My immediate reaction was feeling elated yet mixed with some sense of reality. I went so far as to fantasize that mom who is 92 years old might now live to 100.

My heart previously had been telling me that mom had given up. Once again she has proved me wrong! Or should I say knowing all too well, that this "rebirth" may only last for a day, month, or year until mom can no longer go on.

While I am on this whirlwind I cannot help but feel the bumps and curves as Alzheimer's continues to speed along its tracks. There are so many times I wish for this ride to come to an end.

Why am I not fully able to go with the flow? Am I prepared for this roller coaster ride? I know that I am not being a pessimist. Could it be that I am just being a realist? How silly that I not want mom to have "good "days. Of course I do. For some, this may seem like a miracle yet anyone who understands this disease knows it cannot last.

In the world of dementia the patient does not get to win. There is no cure.

THE RIGHT TO LIVE OR DIE
June 13, 2017

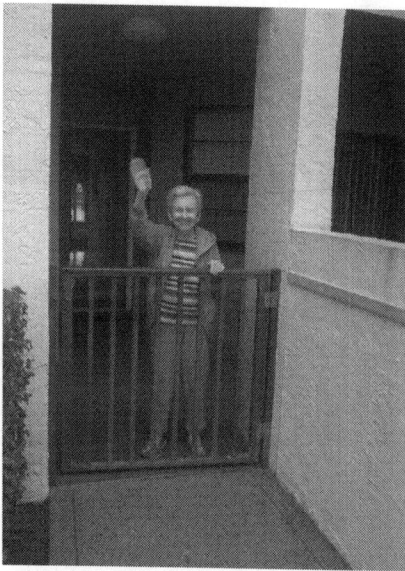

There have been moments when I feel somewhat lost about my deepest feelings regarding my mother. Through these last 14 years as I witnessed her slipping away, I have been able to remain thankful and cherish that she is still alive.

Since her illness I have fallen in love with her unconditionally. At times we shared our laughter and acted so silly almost as if we were teenagers. Today as the disease progresses things with mom are quite different.

My love for her remains undeniable yet when someone in my Alzheimer's Support Group loses their parent my hopeful attitude fades away and thoughts can certainly haunt me. Several weeks ago two members from my group suddenly lost their mothers. It made me wonder why those who joined the group after me, have lost their parents before me; each and every time I question why mom is still alive after having dementia for so many years

What kind of life can mom now possibly have now? She exists, but does she really? Is this life worth living as she no longer has any appreciation of any of the beautiful things that once surrounded her world? Memories of her husband and children are all but gone.

Mom use to love to go to museums, movies and theatre. She enjoyed her morning walks and strolling on the beach. She adored reading, had a great quest for knowledge and loved taking continuing educational classes. For many years none of these things sustain in her life.

Although she probably does not know the difference, she walks around sterile hallways passing others who are confined to wheelchairs and no longer speak. I have often said that she is the lucky one yet I now question....is she? (Since I wrote this mom is in a wheelchair although two aides from restorative therapy come and walk with her each day. They are trying to get her to walk. I have been told that she no longer has the strength nor energy since her illness this past January.)

If she could speak for herself or see herself through different eyes would she want to keep on living? I believe deep in my heart I know her answer. The answer is what I truly would want for myself. Mom will turn 93 years old in August and there have been many years that have come and gone that she has no idea of her age, her life, her family, nor even her existence.

Most of us choose not to speak about this yet it is something that as human beings should be our right. We should be able to make our own choice of how we live and when we should die. My choice has always been with dignity and that is what I so heartily wish for my mother.

Regardless of your beliefs I am certain that we can all agree that Alzheimer's is one of the cruelest diseases. It takes away ones entire world as if it never existed. It has no cure and the ending can be gruesome. So I ask you, should we have the right to choose if we live or die?

MY WISHES
October 8, 2017

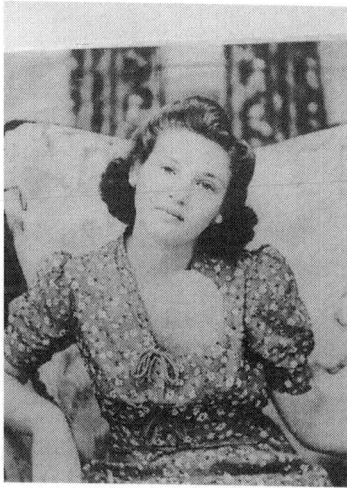

My writings about my journey with my mother have become rather scarce, there is not a day that goes by that I don't think of her. My feelings seem to fluctuate daily from a smile on my face to a pang in my heart about the world she now lives in.

My "lifeline "is being able to contact her nurses several days a week. Each time I ask them to deliver a message to her. Please tell mom that "her daughter Lisa loves her and misses her". They all assure me that they will. Hopefully for one minute mom thinks or remembers me. Either way it makes me feel that we are connecting since I live so far away

I often get questioned about how mom is doing. I know that whoever asks is being both thoughtful and kind yet it is a rather difficult complex question to answer. Considering that mom has Alzheimer's for fourteen years and, is on no medication at the age of 93, I guess one could say, that she is doing well, yet living a life of non-existence.

Last January mom became so ill that we put her on hospice and thought she would pass away. I actually prayed each day that this would happen. I stopped praying since my prayers were not answered and somehow she "bounced" back.

Mom was taken off of hospice and is now confined to a wheelchair. Sadly she no longer has the strength or maybe know-how to walk. Her days of walking around in her Merry Walker have come to a halt. Mostly she sits with her eyes closed and every once in a while she "perks" up and says something. When the aides or the nurses interact with her she somewhat, responds yet, that is pretty much the extent of her life. I know mom would no longer want to be alive and honestly speaking, neither would I.

Letter To My Mom

I hope that when her time is up she passes away as peacefully and painlessly as possible. How I wish that I could give her this last final gift. I want to hug her and take care of her in a different way than she had ever cared for me. She gave me life, and, how I wish to be able to give her peace.

HONORING OUR MOTHER'S
2018

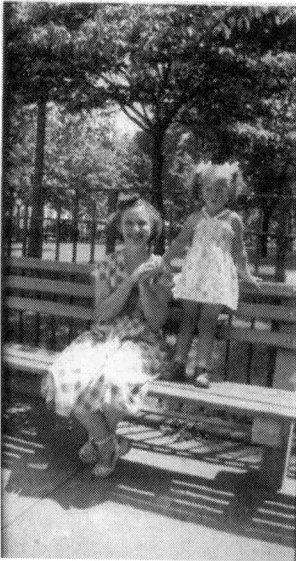

I was asked several years ago to write a letter to my mom which appeared in a book. After reading other letters that also appeared with mine, I realized that I was not the only one, who at one time, had a fractured relationship with their mother. A relationship that needed healing.

Today my relationship is not only healed it is one that I cherish. Mom has taught me so much about life, even when I was unable to recognize it. She is a lady who has given me strength, integrity and what I refer to as "tough" love. Mom was always there for me, and since she has Alzheimer's, my relationship with her for the last fourteen years has changed drastically. It is now one filled with unconditional love.

Being a mother myself I certainly remember when I was pregnant and the day that my son entered the world. I will never forget the birth of my one and only child. I melted as I held him in my arms for the very first time. I was also nervous since this was so brand new to me.

Being a mother is one of the best gifts in the world yet, at times, it can also be challenging. I believe that no matter what your relationship is, or was, with your mother, that when you look deep into your heart you can feel the love.

I have a friend who recently lost her mother. After her mother passed away I listened to what she had to say, which came down to that she loved her, no matter what transpired between the two of them.

How lovely it would be for all of us to celebrate our Mother's. Here is my letter:

LETTER TO MY MOM MY HERO
June 17, 2015

Mom, as I sit down to write my letter I wonder how I can possibly start to share all my feelings with you. So much has changed since you developed Alzheimer's 11 years ago. As I gather my thoughts I realize that you will not be able to comprehend most of what I say.

As a teenager I loved you, yet somehow I wanted one of my friend's mothers to be my mother. Then, after you became ill I fell so deeply in love with you. An unconditional love was born and since then you have inspired me each and every day.

I'm not really sure why my sentiments changed so drastically, I just know that I was given a second chance to feel a deep love and appreciation for you. As I reflect back through these years you have inspired me and have become my hero.

Your humor, your smiles, your sweetness have melted my heart. In several months you will be turning 91 years "young". You can still be feisty and, as you run around in your Merry Walker, I wonder what you could possibly be thinking. Of course I could ask you, yet as silly as that might seem you would not be able to remember anything.

Before entering the nursing home over two years ago, I spoke to you every single day. We ended each call throwing each other our kisses. I have continued to phone the nursing home every day only wanting to hear how you are doing. On occasion I get lucky and am able to hear your sweet voice.

Most of the time you say hello, and after a minute you just drop the phone. You do not even realize that I called or recognize the sound of my voice. Recently I was able to catch you when you were having a minute of clarity. You sounded free of Alzheimer's as you shared that you missed me. These words immediately melted my heart. After hanging up the phone I knew that this was a magical moment, an occasion for me to treasure.

Mom, I am also a mother. My son, your only grandchild is 27 years old. You adored him and yet today you no longer remember who he is. There have been times that you think you have seven children and days when you think you have none. As a mother I cannot envision that one day I might also not know that I have a child.

I find it hard to believe that a disease like this can wipe away your whole world as if it never existed, leaving your mind a blank canvas. Daddy passed away almost twenty two years ago and I do not believe that you have much recollection of him. I'm actually happy that he is no longer alive. I cannot imagine the pain he would have endured watching you fade away.

Today, in your world, I would have to help you brush your teeth, comb your hair, eat your food and get dressed. As a child you once did all of this for me, as well as comforting me when I was sick, or perhaps feeling a little blue. Yet with everything that has changed, at least I know that we still have each other to share our love.

What has changed is that our roles have reversed. Now it is my turn to care for you as you once cared for me. The truth is mom that no matter whatever you can or cannot do, I am still your daughter and you will always be my mother.

Life is strange; for out of you becoming ill I have discovered a whole new world. I was given a second chance to love you unconditionally. You have opened my heart to such a deep compassionate love. Mom as I end my letter, I just want to share with you, how very much I adore you. I feel honored and I am so proud that you are my mother.

Your one and only daughter,

Lisa

Update:
Mom has Alzheimer's for 14+ years and is now 93 years old and has been living in the nursing home for over 5 years.
My father passed away July 28, 1995.
My son Logan is now 30 years old.
Mom is now confined to a wheelchair and is doing "good'.

Book- My Mom My Hero; Alzheimer's
Available from Amazon.com and other retailers

Letter To My Mom

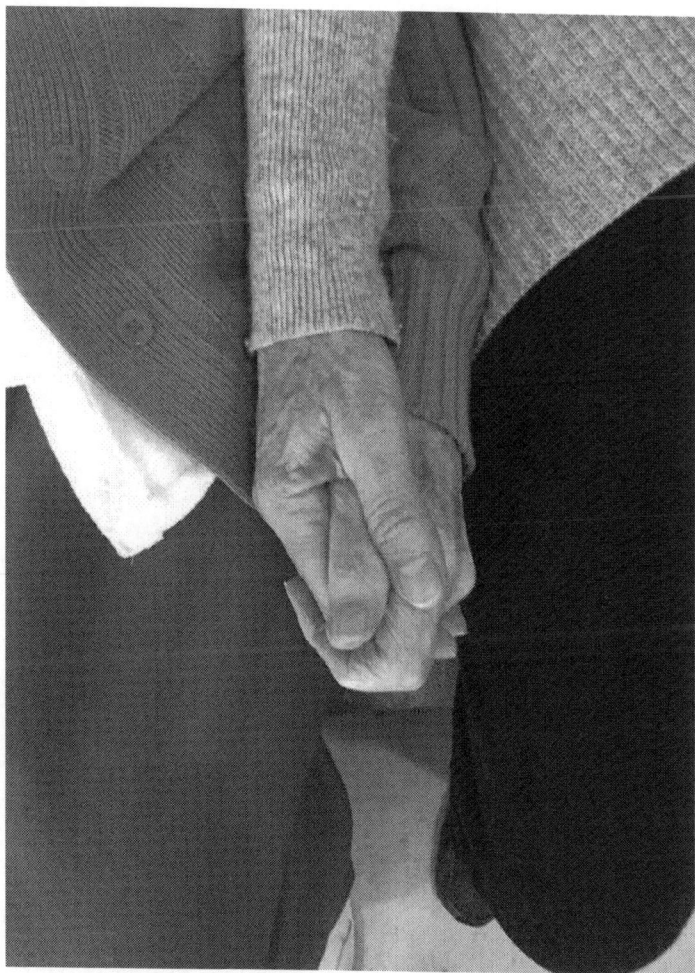

Made in the USA
Lexington, KY
03 April 2018